The Forgotten Aged:
Ethnic, Psychiatric,
and Societal Minorities

The Forgotten Aged: Ethnic, Psychiatric, and Societal Minorities

T. L. Brink, PhD
Editor

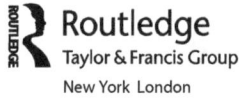

Routledge
Taylor & Francis Group
New York London

First published 1993 by The Haworth Press, Inc.

Published 2020 by Routledge
605 Third Avenue, New York, NY 10017
2 Park Square, Milton Park, Abingdon, Oxon OX14 4RN

First issued in paperback 2021

Routledge is an imprint of the Taylor & Francis Group, an informa business

Copyright © 1993 Taylor & Francis

The Forgotten Aged: Ethnic, Psychiatric, and Societal Minorities has also been published as *Clinical Gerontologist*, Volume 14, Number 1 1993.

Library of Congress Cataloging-in-Publication Data

The Forgotten aged: ethnic, psychiatric, and societal minorities/T.L. Brink, editor.
    p. # cm.
    "Has also been published as Clinical gerontologist, volume 14, number 1, 1993"–T.p. verso
    Includes bibliographical references and index.
    ISBN 1-56024-572-7 (alk. paper)
    1. Aged–Mental health services–United States. 2. Minority aged–Mental health services–
    United States. 3. Social work with the aged–United States. I. Brink, T.L. (Terry L.)
RC451.4.A5F67 1993   93-40823
362.1'9897'008693–dc20   CIP

ISBN 13: 978-1-138-98927-6 (pbk)
ISBN 13: 978-1-56024-572-8 (hbk)
ISBN 13: 978-1-315-82533-5 (ebk)

DOI: 10.4324/9781315825335

The Forgotten Aged: Ethnic, Psychiatric, and Societal Minorities

CONTENTS

ABOUT THE EDITOR

T. L. Brink, PhD, is currently on the faculty of Crafton Hills College in Yucaipa, California, and Loma Linda University. He is a member of the International Council of Psychologists, the International Psychogeriatric Association, the National Social Science Association, the Western Psychological Association, and the Midwestern Psychological Association. The American Psychological Association named him a Distinguished Visitor in 1984.

During his career, Dr. Brink has developed the International Version of the Mental Status Questionnaire, the Geriatric Depression Scale, the Hypochondriasis Scale (Institutional Geriatric), the Scale for Paranoia (Observer Rated Geriatric), and the Stimulus Recognition Test. His books include *Geriatric Psychotherapy* (Human Sciences Press, 1979; Imago, 1983); *The Middle Class Credo* (R&E, 1984; Fawcett Gold Medal, 1985); *Clinical Gerontology: A Guide to Assessment and Intervention* (The Haworth Press, Inc., 1986); *The Elderly Uncooperative Patient* (The Haworth Press, Inc., 1987); *Mental Health in the Nursing Home* (The Haworth Press Inc., 1990); and *Hispanic Aged Mental Health* (The Haworth Press, Inc., 1992). He has published over 300 articles, chapters and reviews. Dr. Brink has been the editor of the journal *Clinical Gerontologist* since 1982.

Introduction

This book began as a special volume for *Clinical Gerontologist*. We have previously published several articles, clinical comments, and book reviews about ethnic minorities, including a booklength special volume, *Hispanic Aged Mental Health*. We have also published on some of the special topics contained in these chapters. However, it has become apparent to me that there are some elders who have received the lion's share of our attention: dementia patients and their caregivers. While this focus can be justified by the widespread and severe nature of late life organic brain syndrome, it should not excuse ignoring other sorts of problems. Similarly, most of the case studies we have published and most of the subjects in the research we have previously cited have been of European-American extraction (white), married or widowed, living in urban or suburban areas, and had some adult children who could be consulted. The purpose of this volume is to explore the mental health concerns of elders who do not fit into these paradigms: the forgotten aged.

TLB

[Haworth co-indexing entry note]: "Introduction." Brink, T. L. Co-published simultaneously in *Clinical Gerontologist* (The Haworth Press, Inc.) Vol. 14, No. 1, 1993, p. 1; and: *The Forgotten Aged: Ethnic, Psychiatric, and Societal Minorities* (ed: T. L. Brink) The Haworth Press, Inc., 1993, p. 1. Multiple copies of this article/chapter may be purchased from The Haworth Document Delivery Center. Call 1-800-3-HAWORTH (1-800-342-9678) between 9:00 - 5:00 (EST) and ask for DOCUMENT DELIVERY CENTER.

SECTION ONE: ASSESSMENT OF ETHNIC MINORITIES

Chapter One

Use of the Mini-Mental State Examination in African American Elders

F. M. Baker, MD, MPH
Beverly H. Robinson, PhD, RN, C
Bess Stewart, PhD, RN, CS

Editor's Introduction

Baker, Robinson and Stewart investigated whether a commonly used screening test for dementia, Folstein's Mini-Mental Status Exam is useful with African Americans. The sample was comprised of African American elders (n = 55) with a mean age of 78 years, and was 90% female. Subjects consented to be

F. M. Baker is Associate Professor, Department of Psychiatry, University of Maryland at Baltimore. Beverly H. Robinson is Associate Professor and Bess Stewart is Assistant Professor, Department of Nursing at University of Texas Health Science, San Antonio, TX.

The authors wish to acknowledge the contribution of Richard Hebel, Professor of Biostatistics, Department of Epidemiology and Preventive Medicine, University of Maryland at Baltimore for his invaluable assistance with data analysis.

This work was completed with the assistance of funding from the National Institute of Mental Health, Grant No. 2K07 MH00816-02.

[Haworth co-indexing entry note]: "Use of the Mini-Mental State Examination in African American Elders." Baker, F. M., Beverly H. Robinson, and Bess Stewart. Co-published simultaneously in *Clinical Gerontologist* (The Haworth Press, Inc.) Vol. 14, No. 1, 1993, pp. 5-13; and: *The Forgotten Aged: Ethnic, Psychiatric, and Societal Minorities* (ed: T. L. Brink) The Haworth Press, Inc., 1993, pp. 5-13. Multiple copies of this article/chapter may be purchased from The Haworth Document Delivery Center. Call 1-800-3-HAWORTH (1-800-342-9678) between 9:00 - 5:00 (EST) and ask for DOCUMENT DELIVERY CENTER.

screened with the MMSE, and a week later were given a comprehensive psychiatric evaluation. Using an MMSE cut-off score of under 24 as indicative of cognitive impairment, 18% of this sample fell into that category. Using the psychiatric exam as the standard of comparison, the MMSE had a sensitivity of 70% and a specificity of 93%.

INTRODUCTION

The assessment of cognitive function among African American populations has received increasing attention in the recent literature.[1-6] Demographic studies of the United States population[7,8] have projected that older African Americans will comprise 70% of the minority elderly by 2030. The fastest growing segment of the older, black population is the old-old, i.e., persons age 85 and older.[6,7]

Several authors have reported on the limitations of the Mini-Mental State Examination[9-11] as a screening instrument. The widespread use of the Mini-Mental State Examination (MMSE) has resulted in establishing it as an international standard for the assessment of cognitive function.[12,13] Specific problems identified with the use of the MMSE include an increased rate of false positives in persons with less than an 8th grade education.[6, 9-11] Escobar et al.[9] found that Hispanic Americans in Los Angeles had increased problems with three specific areas: retrograde spelling of the word, "world," serial subtraction of 7 beginning with 100, and the interpretation of the phrase–"no ifs, ands, or buts."

Although 25% of older African Americans in the current cohort of elders completed a college education, the majority of these elders had less formal education. Several investigators have documented the interaction of educational level and MMSE scores. Persons with less than an eighth grade education were found to have lower scores on the MMSE. If the MMSE is used to screen populations of African American elders for cognitive impairment, persons with a lower educational level could be identified incorrectly as having cognitive impairment who do not. The issue of language will be of an increasing concern as the number of persons of African Caribbean heritage increases in the black American population.[14] The data from the

Hispanic population of Los Angeles[9] demonstrated the importance of language as a variable in the interpretation of the results of screening instruments that assess cognitive function.

This study reports on the use of the MMSE in a population of community resident African American elders. The focus of this study was two-fold: (1) to assess the specific problems or concerns involved in using the MMSE in this population and (2) to establish whether educational level affected the observed MMSE scores.

METHODOLOGY

The sample was drawn from two sites in the city of San Antonio, Texas: a senior citizen housing complex, and a senior center. The senior housing complex was comprised of 72 apartments in two-story dwellings located in a section of the city that was predominantly African American. The senior center was located in the same area. In addition to providing hot meals, health screening programs, and various community activities, it also provided the opportunity for volunteer activities.

The Department of Nursing of the University of Texas Health Science Center at San Antonio had established linkages with these settings over several years. These senior sites served as locations for the community health rotations for graduate nursing students. When the community boards of each setting were approached to obtain permission to contact their members concerning participation in the study, approval was readily granted. The research team was comprised of African American investigators: two native Texan nursing faculty with Ph.D.'s (BVH & BS), and one geriatric psychiatrist, a resident of Texas for two years (FMB).

All consenting African American elders in the two sites were screened by two of the investigators (BVH & BS). The screening battery was comprised of the MMSE, the 15-item Geriatric Depression Scale, the Hamilton Depression Scale, and a background informational sheet that obtained basic demographic information (age, sex, race, marital status, and educational attainment), current medical problems, and current medications.

Within an average of seven days of the initial screening, the 55 African American elders who comprised the sample completed a comprehensive psychiatric evaluation. Only three interviews were not completed in this time period due to a conflict in volunteer work (N = 1) and a planned vacation by two study participants (N = 2). The psychiatrist (FMB) completing the psychiatric evaluation was blind to the results of the screening. The results of the depression screening instruments are presented in another publication.[15]

RESULTS

The sample was composed of 41 females and 14 males; 74% of the sample was female. Utilizing the original threshold score of 23 or lower as evidence of cognitive impairment, 18% of the sample (N = 10) were identified as having evidence of cognitive impairment (screening positive). The mean age of this subsample was 78 and ninety percent were female.

When the sample was divided into those screening positive and negative for cognitive impairment, the mean age and mean MMSE scores are shown in Table 1. The differences between mean MMSE score and mean age were not statistically significant. There was no statistically significant difference between the genders on mean MMSE scores. Of the 45 subjects who screened negative on the MMSE, only 5 (11%) were identified as having a psychiatric disorder. These diagnoses included: Major Depression (N = 1), Bipolar Disorder, Manic (N = 1), Adjustment Disorder with Mixed Emotional Features (N = 1), and Organic Mood Disorder due to Hypothyroidism (N = 1).

Ten subjects (18%) screened positive on the MMSE. Table 2

Table 1:   Comparison of Mean Age and Mean Mini-Mental State
            Examination (MMSE) Scores Between African American
            Elders Screening Positive and African American Elders
            Screening Negative

MMSE Screening Results	Mean MMSE Score	Mean Age
Positive (N=10)	20	78
Negative (N=32)	28	75

Fisher's exact test, 2 tailed = 1.000;
not statistically significant

Table 2:   Educational Levels Compared with Mini-Mental State Score
            (MMSE) Among Elders Screening Positive on the MMSE
            (Evidence of Cognitive Impairment) N = 10

Subject	MMSE Score	Education Grades Completed	DSM III R Diagnosis
80 BF	15	00	290.00
70 BF	17	12	296.41
74 BF	18	11	296.25
77 BM	21	00	296.22
72 BF	21	05	V62.89
75 BF	21	11	V71.09
76 BF	23	07	296.24
81 BF	23	12	309.00
85 BF	23	11	V71.09
89 BF	23	02	V71.09

Correlation coefficient (r) not statistically
significant. T=.0000, 8 df, p=1.000

summarizes the MMSE scores, educational level, and DSM-III-R diagnoses for those elders who had evidence of cognitive impairment on the MMSE. When a correlation coefficient was calculated to establish whether MMSE scores increased or decreased as educational level increased, the correlation value was zero, indicating the absence of a linear relationship. There was also no statistical significance between the two groups: t = .0000, 8 df, p = 1.000.

When African American elders identified as having cognitive impairment by MMSE were compared with elders identified by the psychiatric evaluation as having cognitive impairment, there was a statistically significant difference between the two groups (Fisher's exact test, 2 tailed = .0001). The MMSE identified 3 patients of the ten with psychiatric disorders (30%) as having cognitive impairment who were intact by psychiatric evaluation, the reference standard. The MMSE, also, found 3 patients of the 45 without psychiatric disorders (7%) as having cognitive impairment.

When the number of elders correctly identified as having cognitive impairment was evaluated, the sensitivity was 70% and the specificity was 93% in this sample.

DISCUSSION

Although the majority of African American elders have been shown by national statistics to be predominantly single women who are below the poverty level,[16] the heterogeneity of the older, black population has been emphasized by several authors.[8,17-19] The population of elders identified from two senior citizen sites in San Antonio, Texas provided specific data illustrating this heterogeneity. The educational level of this sample is consistent with data from the National Center on Health Statistics[20] that reports that 25% of older, African Americans have completed college. The 29% of this sample that completed 13 to 18 years of education beyond high school were employed in state government positions, were teachers, and managed their own businesses. In this convenience sample the MMSE proved to be a modestly effective screening instrument with a sensitivity of 70% and a specificity of 93%. Confirming reports in the literature,[21-24] African American elders with mood disorders and dementia all had evidence of cognitive impairment by results of the MMSE. These findings of cognitive impairment were consistent with the clinical evaluation. When MMSE scores and grades of education completed were compared among those elders with psychiatric disorders, MMSE scores did not vary with educational attainment. This result was surprising in view of the existing literature. Although education varied from 00 to 12 years in this subsample, the MMSE scores, which ranged from 15 to 23, were not found to correlate with the grades of education completed.

Among those African American elders without psychiatric disorder, those who screened positive on the MMSE had completed only an elementary education and were older (over age 80). Education and age were confounded because older African Americans were more likely to have completed less formal education. Although inter-rater reliability in the administration of the instruments was established, these findings will need to be replicated by other studies in larger, population-based samples. The MMSE may be less useful in community-based elders without psychiatric illness. This has implications for the screening of community-resident populations in which a variety of levels of educational attainment will be found among African American elders.

The presence of undiagnosed psychiatric disorders in this sample is an important finding. Although the issue of misdiagnosis of psychiatric disorders among African American populations has been addressed and a growing body of literature has presented specific case examples, this is one of the first studies to screen and evaluate a sample of African American elders for the presence of psychiatric disorders. Although some of these elders joked about needing to see a "head doctor" about the "trouble in their lives," the majority of those with specific psychiatric disorders did *not* report the usual pattern of symptoms. They did not present the traditional "chief complaints" of depressed patients. Instead these elders reported that they would "not be doing well" if it was not for "their faith in God." They were able to handle "problems" because they knew "that God wouldn't give me more than I could bear." When asked if they felt sad, blue, or down, they stated that "I've had some trouble" or "It's been hard." They followed their report of "problems/troubles" of concern with such statements as "I know that it'll get better some day" and "He (God) has always been there for me." Only when extensive probing was done did some report of the neurovegetative symptoms of depression by DSM-III-R criteria emerge.

If these findings are replicated in larger, population based samples of African American elders they would suggest that the MMSE may be a useful screening instrument for African American elders with minimal formal education who have psychiatric disorders, but less useful in non-psychiatrically ill, community resident elders. In addition to providing further data on the use of the MMSE in a sample of older, black Americans, our work provides specific information on the presentation of depressive illness in African American elders.

With the changing demographic profile of the older population in the United States, it will be important to understand the specific presentation of disorders as well as the most effective and efficient manner of their identification in this population of ethnic elders. The recent work of the Task Force on Ethnic Diagnosis as part of the DSM-IV Task Force[25] has provided an important summary of research concerns for the specific population of ethnic minorities. This report addresses issues of diagnosis and treatment and its publication should stimulate further research in this area.

REFERENCES

1. Schoenberg, B.S., Anderson, D.W., & Haerer, A.F. (1985). Severe dementia. Prevalence and clinical features in a biracial U.S. population. *Archives of Neurology 42*, 740-743.

2. Folstein, M., Anthony, J.C., Parhard, J., Duffy, B., & Gruenberg, E.M. (1985). The meaning of cognitive impairment in the elderly. *Journal of the American Geriatric Society 33*, 228-235.

3. Fillenbaum, G., Heyman, A., Williams, K., & Prosnitz, B. (1990). Sensitivity and specificity of standardized screens of cognitive impairment and dementia among elderly black and white community residents. *Journal of Clinical Epidemiology 43*, 651-660.

4. Baker, F.M. (1991). Dementing illness in African American populations: evaluation and management for the primary physician. *Journal of Geriatric Psychiatry 24*, 73-91.

5. Heyman, A., Fillenbaum, G., Prosnitz, B., Raiford, K., Burchett, B., & Clark, C. (1991). Estimated prevalence of dementia among elderly black and white community residents. *Archives of Neurology 48*, 594-598.

6. Folstein, M.F., Bassett, S.S., Anthony, J.C., Romanoski, A.J., & Nestadt, G.R. (1991). Dementia: case ascertainment in a community survey. *Journal of Gerontology 46*, M132-M138.

7. Manual, R.C. (1988). The demography of older blacks. In *The Black Physical and Psychosocial Health* (pp. 25-49). New York: Springer Publishing Company.

8. Gibson, R. (1986). *Blacks in An Aging Society.* New York: Carnegie Corporation.

9. Escobar, J.I., Burnam, M.A., Karno, M., Forsythe, A., Landsverk, J., & Golding, J.M. (1986). Use of the Mini-Mental State Examination (MMSE) in a community population of mixed ethnicity: cultural and linguistic artifacts. *Journal of Nervous and Mental Disorders 17*, 607-614.

10. Roca, R.P., Klein, L.E., Kirby, S.M., McArthur, J.C., Vogelsang, G.B., Folstein, M.F., & Smith, C.R. (1984). Recognition of dementia among medical patients. *Archives of Internal Medicine 144*, 73-75.

11. Baker, F.M. (1989). Screening instruments for cognitive impairment. *Hospital and Community Psychiatry 40*, 339-340.

12. Rocca, W.A., Amaducci, L.A., & Schoenberg, B.S. (1986). Epidemiology of clinically diagnosed Alzheimer's Disease. *Annals of Neurology 19*, 415-424.

13. Li, G., Shen, Y.C., Chen, C.H., Zhau, Y.W., Li, S.R., & Lu, M. (1991). A three-year follow-up study of age-related dementia in an urban area of Beijing. *Acta Psychiatrica Scandinavica 83*, 99-104.

14. Allen, E.A. (1988). West Indians. In *Clinical Guidelines in Cross-Cultural Mental Health* (pp. 305-333). L. Comas-Dia, & E.E.H. Griffith (Eds.). New York: John Wiley & Sons.

15. Baker, F.M., Robinson, B.S., & Stewart, B. (in press). Sensitivity and specificity of the 15-item Geriatric Depression Scale in African American elders. *Journal of Geriatric Psychiatry and Neurology*.

16. Gottlieb, G. (1991). Financial issues. In *Comprehensive Review of Geriatric Psychiatry* (pp. 667-686). J. Sadavoy, L.W. Lazarus, & L.F. Javik (Eds.). Washington, DC: American Psychiatric Press.

17. Jackson, J.S. (1991). *Life in Black America*. Newbury Park, CA: Sage Publications.

18. Wilkerson, C.B., & Spurlock, J. (1986). The mental health of black Americans. In *Ethnic Psychiatry* (pp. 13-60). C.B. Wilkerson (Ed.). New York: Plenum Medical Book Company.

19. Baker, F.M. (1992). Ethnic minority elders: a mental health research agenda. *Hospital and Community Psychiatry 43*, 337-338.

20. National Center on Health Statistics. (1991). *Health. United States, 1990*. Washington DC: U.S. Government Printing Office.

21. Heisel, M.A., & Faulkner, A. (1982). Religiosity in an older black population. *The Gerontologist 22*, 354-358.

22. Taylor, R.J. (1986). Religious participation among elderly blacks. *The Gerontologist 26*, 630-636.

23. Taylor, R.J. (1988). Structural determinants of religious participation among black Americans. *Review of Religious Research 30*, 114-125.

24. Taylor, R.J., & Chatters L.M. (1988). Church members as a source of informal social support. *Review of Religious Research 30*, 193-203.

25. Mezzich, J.E., Kleinman, A., Fabrega, H., Good, B., Johnson-Powell, G., Lin, K.M., Manson, S., & Parron, D. (1992). *Cultural Proposals for DSM-IV*. Pittsburgh, PA: University of Pittsburgh.

16. Sue, S., Allen, D.B. & Conaway, L. (1978). The responsiveness and equality of mental health care to Chicanos and Native Americans.

17. Snowden, L.R. & Cheung, F.K. (1990). Use of inpatient mental health services by members of ethnic minority groups. *American Psychologist*, 45, 347–355.

18. Spielberger, C.D., Gorsuch, R.L. & Lushene, R.E. (1970). *Manual for the State-Trait Anxiety Inventory.* Palo Alto: Consulting Psychologists Press.

19. Sue, S., Fujino, D.C., Hu, L., Takeuchi, D.T. & Zane, N.W.S. (1991). Community mental health services for ethnic minority groups: a test of the cultural responsiveness hypothesis. *Journal of Consulting and Clinical Psychology*, 59, 533–540.

20. Snowden, L.R. & Cheung, F.K. (1990).

21. Takeuchi, D.T., Sue, S. & Yeh, M. (1995).

22. Vernon, S.W. & Roberts, R.E. (1982).

23. Vega, W.A. & Rumbaut, R.G. (1991).

24. Williams, D.R. (1990).

25. Zane, N., Sue, S. & Hu, L. (1991).

Chapter Two

Assessing Depressive Symptoms in African American and Mexican American Elders

F. M. Baker, MD, MPH
David V. Espino, MD
Beverly H. Robinson, PhD, RN, C
Bess Stewart, PhD, RN, CS

Editor's Introduction

Now the same mental health researchers add Espino to their team and report on their investigation in assessing a different mental disorder, depression, this time with both African-Ameri-

F. M. Baker is Associate Professor, Department of Psychiatry, University of Maryland at Baltimore. David V. Espino is Assistant Professor, Department of Family Practice, University of Texas Health Science Center at San Antonio. Beverly H. Robinson is Associate Professor and Bess Stewart is Assistant Professor, Department of Nursing, University of Texas Health Science Center, San Antonio.

This study was completed with support provided by NIMH Grant Number 2 K07 MH00816-02 and Subgrant A8 from the South Texas Health Research Center.

[Haworth co-indexing entry note]: "Assessing Depressive Symptoms in African American and Mexican American Elders." Baker, F. M. et al. Co-published simultaneously in *Clinical Gerontologist* (The Haworth Press, Inc.) Vol. 14, No. 1, 1993, pp. 15-29; and: *The Forgotten Aged: Ethnic, Psychiatric, and Societal Minorities* (ed: T. L. Brink) The Haworth Press, Inc., 1993, pp. 15-29. Multiple copies of this article/chapter may be purchased from The Haworth Document Delivery Center. Call 1-800-3-HAWORTH (1-800- 342-9678) between 9:00 - 5:00 (EST) and ask for DOCUMENT DELIVERY CENTER.

15

cans (n = 58) in the community and Mexican-Americans (n = 57) with affective disorder. While I have used the GDS with both populations, and believe it to be the most appropriate test for depression screening, the research reported here raises some questions about the scale's sensitivity: particularly the ability to pick out major depressive disorder from other affective disorders.

INTRODUCTION

Recent literature has begun the description of major depressive illness in older American populations (Gurland, 1976; Weissman, 1981; Ruess et al., 1988; Alexopoulos et al., 1988; Cassem, 1988; Neighbors et al., 1989; Baker et al., 1992; NIH Concensus Conference on Depression, 1992). The symptoms, course of illness, and outcomes of depression with and without treatment are being studied by several teams of investigators. The recent NIH Consensus Conference on Depression in Older Patients (1992) summarized the existing knowledge and emphasized the number of areas where more rigorously designed investigations were needed. Specific areas highlighted included the study of specifically detailed populations of patients meeting DSM III-R criteria for Major Depressive Disorder, the need for well-designed studies of specific psychopharmacologic agents in specific subpopulations of the elderly, and the organization of methodologically sound studies of the outcome of specific psychotherapeutic modalities in the treatment of depression.

Although older Americans through the 1980s were predominately white, this pattern will change over the next 40 years (Angel & Hogen, 1989). By 2030 twenty-five percent of U.S. residents age 65 and older will be non-white, combining the populations of older African Americans, American Indians and Alaska Natives, Asian Americans and Pacific Islanders, and Hispanic Americans. By 2030 the majority of persons age 85 and older will be ethnic minority elders. This changing demographic profile of the U.S. population requires that mental health professionals expand their knowledge and understanding of these populations.

Several authors have suggested that Major Depressive Disorder may present in a different manner among persons of different ethnic backgrounds (Gurland, 1976; Smith-Ruiz, 1985; Mezzich, 1992). Among depressed African Americans, Asian Americans, and Hispanic Americans, an increased report of somatic complaints (headache, stomach ache, backache, pain and chronic fatigue) has been reported. In studies of some Native American tribes the presentation of depression was conceptualized as a disharmony with nature, a complaint consistent with the tribes' conceptualization of the relationship of man and nature (Baker & Lightfoot, 1993). Rather than a report of a blue or sad mood, the Japanese describe a depressed mood in terms of a "storm" (Sakauye et al., 1993).

Several instruments have been developed to screen persons for the presence of depressive symptoms (Hamilton, 1960; Beck et al., 1961; Sung, 1965; Roberts et al., 1981). The Geriatric Depression Scale (GDS) was the most recent instrument that was developed specifically to screen the elderly for depression (Yesavage & Brink, 1983). Neurovegetative signs increase with medical illnesses and the side effect of medications. Because the elderly have at least 3 active medical problems and take at least 3.6 medications per day, questions on neurovegetative signs were eliminated from the GDS.

Originally developed as a 30-item screening instrument (Yesavage & Brink, 1983), the GDS was modified to a 15-item instrument (Sheikh & Yesavage, 1986). Various studies have utilized either the 30-item or the 15-item version. Further, a Spanish translation of the GDS was completed and used in a few studies. Brink (1992) questioned the efficacy of the 30-item GDS in Mexican American elders and found it to be of somewhat limited usefulness because it deleted somatic symptoms which were the major complaint in his sample of depressed Mexican Americans.

The Hamilton Depression Scale (HDS) has been utilized in the majority of studies of depressive disorder (Hamilton, 1960). International and national collaborative studies of depression have utilized the HDS as the screening instrument for entry into the study. It has been used, also, to show improvement in depressive symptoms following treatment. The Beck Depression Inventory, a self-report scale of depressive symptoms (BDI), has been used effectively in a few Native American tribes and with African American populations of mixed age (Manson et al., 1987, Rosenthal et al., 1987).

The Center for Epidemiologic Studies of Depression Scale (CES-D) was developed by the Epidemiology Section of the National Institute of Mental Health (CES-D) specifically to screen populations of community residents for the presence of depressive symptoms. The majority of epidemiologic studies which screened mixed-age, community-resident, African Americans for depressive symptoms used the CES-D (Brown, 1990). A specific concern with this instrument was the need to use a higher threshold for the designation of depressive symptoms reflecting depressive illness; i.e., a score of 18 versus 16. Because of the mortality among African Americans secondary to multiple, chronic medical illnesses and the side effects of medications, community resident, African Americans were likely to screen positive on the CES-D with a threshold of 16 (Murrell et al., 1986). In a study of 5 American Indian tribes the CES-D was found to be a reliable and valid test to screen for depressive symptoms in these tribes (Manson et al., 1987). Cronbach's alpha was .86 which indicated very good internal consistency and measurement of depression (Barón et al., In Press).

When the Health Opinion Survey was used to screen a subsample of Santa Clara County, CA residents for psychoneurosis, level of acculturation was found to be a factor that influenced the report of symptoms (Vega et al., 1985). Mexican Americans who were Spanish-speaking reported higher rates of psychiatric symptoms in comparison to English-speaking Mexican Americans. The lowest rates of symptoms were reported by whites (Vega et al., 1985). Data from the Los Angeles site of the Epidemiologic Catchment Area Survey were conflicted (Burnam et al., 1987). In this sample higher acculturation was associated with a higher lifetime prevalence of phobias, alcohol abuse or dependence, drug abuse or dependence, major depression or dysthymia with rates higher for native-born, Mexican Americans versus immigrant Mexican Americans. Specific tests to assess the impact of administration of the structured interview in English or Spanish were completed. There were no significant differences in the prevalence of psychiatric disorders based upon the language of interview (Spanish versus English).

This was true whether the study subjects had a median level of acculturation, were recent immigrants, or had been resident in the U.S. for 20 years or more (Burnam et al., 1987).

The CES-D Scale was found to be a reliable instrument. In a later study by Roberts et al. (1989) a bilingual assessment instrument was developed by the research team to determine language preference. Language preference has been used as one indicator of level of acculturation (Mezzich et al., 1992). These authors found no effect of language or ethnic status in the CES-D in their sample of Mexican American and white, psychiatric in-patients and psychiatric outpatients. The CES-D was administered to a sample of community resident Mexican Americans (Aneshensel et al., 1983). It was found to be a valid and reliable instrument in the sample. Level of acculturation and immigrant status were not determined by these authors. In this sample the CES-D had a high sensitivity for depressive and anxiety symptoms and did not discriminate between symptoms of depression, dysthymia, and generalized anxiety. Roberts et al. (1989) questioned whether the CES-D instrument was best conceptualized as a measure of discrimination because it did not discriminate between major depressive disorder and generalized anxiety disorder in their sample.

METHODOLOGY

African American Sample (Community Residents). African American faculty in the School of Nursing of the University of Texas Health Science Center at San Antonio had established a relationship with older African Americans resident in a senior citizen complex. The complex contained 72 apartment units that were built in 1985. These residents were contacted and invited to participate in the study. An additional source of community resident, African American elders was identified from a senior citizen center that served the black community of San Antonio, Texas. This community center served a daily population of 120 elders.[1]

The community board of the senior citizen housing complex and

---

1. The program included a hot luncheon meal, health screening programs, and opportunities for volunteer work within the center.

the Board of Directors of the Senior Citizen Center approved the study and authorized the research team to contact their residents and members. These African American elders were screened by culturally sensitive, African American, doctorally prepared psychiatric nurses who were native Texans familiar with the region. The psychiatric interviews were completed by an African American psychiatrist who was resident in the region for two years. A detailed discussion of the methodology for the African American sample is presented in another paper (Baker et al., 1992).

Mexican American Sample (In-Patient Sample). The Lutheran General Hospital is a 325 bed, general hospital located in the Mexican American community of San Antonio, Texas. It serves a population of 150,000. It contains a 32-bed, in-patient psychiatric unit that is staffed by bilingual psychiatrists and nursing personnel. The director of the in-patient unit at the time of this study in 1988 was a board-certified, San Antonio born, Mexican American psychiatrist who was board certified in psychiatry and a San Antonio native familiar with the Mexican American Community.

In order to establish the validity and reliability of the GDS-S among Mexican American elders and in view of the results with the 15-item GDS in the community-resident, African American sample, it was decided to begin with a sample of Mexican American elders with known DSM-III-R diagnoses of affective disorder. In this sample the presence of depressive symptoms should be identified, readily, provided that the GDS-S was an effective screening instrument for depressive symptoms in this population. Following required approvals by the Institutional Review Board of Lutheran General Hospital and the Director of the in-patient unit, all patients with a diagnosis of affective disorder who were age 55 and older were approached to participate in the study. All those who consented were screened with a Spanish translation of GDS-15 administered by Mexican American, San Antonio-born retirees who were members of the San Antonio chapter of the American Association of Retired Persons (AARP). These AARP volunteers were bilingual, conversant with the regional Mexican American culture, and completed training that established inter-rater reliability at 0.96 for the administration of the GDS-S.

The GDS-15 was translated into Spanish by a team composed of a Mexican American, San Antonio-born, family practice physician (DVE) and a Mexican-American, San Antonio-born, Assistant Professor of Romanic Languages. This translation was reviewed by the AARP volunteers who completed a translation from English to Spanish. A back translation into English was completed to confirm that the key concepts of the GDS-S were not distorted and that they were reliably presented. The resulting GDS-S (Spanish translation of the 15-item GDS) was used as the screening instrument for the Mexican-American elderly sample.

RESULTS

African-American Sample

Fifty-five of the 58 (94%) African American elders who consented to participate in the study and were screened with the 15-item GDS completed the psychiatric interview. The sample was composed of 41 women and 14 men with a mean age of 77. Fifty percent of men were married, and 63% of women were widowed. Educational attainment varied with 24% of the sample having completed college and/or having an advanced degree and 25% of the sample with between 0-6 years of formal education. Twenty percent of the sample (11 of 55) were identified as having a psychiatric disorder (Table 1).

The mean GDS score and Hamilton Depression Score (HDS) per diagnostic grouping varied: Affective Disorder (GDS = 6; HDS = 12);

Table 1: African American Elders

DSM-III-R Diagnosis	N	%
Affective Disorder	6	11%
Adjustment Disorder with Depressed Mood	2	4%
Primary Degenerative Dementia of the Alzheimer's Type, Senile Onset	1	2%
Organic Mental Disorder	2	4%
	11	20%

Adjustment Disorder with Depressed Mood (GDS = 3; HDS = 4); Organic Mental Disorder (GDS = 3; HDS = 5). Utilizing the original GDS cut scores of 6 or more as evidence of depressive symptoms, the sensitivity was 35% and the specificity was 100%. When a lower threshold for the presence of depressive symptoms was used (a cut-score of 4), the sensitivity improved to 64% and the specificity was 95%.

Mexican-American Sample

Fifty-seven consecutive admissions to the in-patient psychiatric unit of the general hospital consented to participate in this study. The sample was composed of 23 men (56%) and 18 women (44%) with a median age of 74; an age of 62-98 years. Marital status and education were not abstracted from the clinical records. Table 2 summarizes the types of affective disorders diagnosed in this sample of older Mexican-American psychiatric patients.

The mean GDS-S scores ranged from 1 to 14 among these older, psychiatric patients. Table 3 compares the GDS-S scores between patients with Major Depressive Disorder and those with Other Depressive Disorder with the original GDS scores. Table 4

Table 2: **DSM-III-R, Psychiatric Disorders Diagnosed on Consecutive Admissions of Mexican American Elders to a General Hospital In-Patient Psychiatric Unit**

DSM-III-R Diagnosis	N	%
Major Depressive Disorder[1]	28	68%
Other Depressive Disorders[2]	13*	32%
	41	100%

[1] Included 18 patients with delusional depression

2 Included: 6 patients with Organic Affective Disorders due to stroke, hypothyroidism, B_{12} deficiency, and Parkinson's Disease
2 patients with Bipolar Disorder, Depressed
3 patients with Dysthymic Disorder
2 patients with Major Depressive Disorder with Panic Attacks

Table 3: GD8-S Scores for Mexican-American Elderly Psychiatric Patients with Major Depressive Disorder (MDD) and Other Depressive Disorders (ODD)

ORIGINAL THRESHOLD

GD8-S	MDD		ODD		Total		
	N	%	N	%	N	%	
0-5 Normal	17	61%	3	23%	20	49%	X^2 = 5.05
6-10 Mildly Suggestive of Depression	9	32%	8	62%	17	41%	df = 2
11-15 Strongly Suggestive of Depression	2	7%	2	15%	4	10%	p = .08
Totals	28	100%	13	100%	41	100%	NS[1]

[1]Not Significant

Table 4: GDS-8 Scores for Mexican American Elderly Psychiatric Patients with Major Depression Disorder (MDD) and Other Depressive Disorder (ODD)

REVISED THRESHOLD

GDS-8	MDD		ODD		Total		
	N	%	N	%			
0-3 Normal	7	25%	2	15%	9	22%	$x^2 = 0.48$
4-15 Suggestive of Depression	21	75%	11	85%	38	78%	df = 1
Totals	28	100%	13	100%	41	100%	p = 0.49

Not Significant

compares the two groups with the revised threshold. When these two groups were combined, a sensitivity of 49% with the original threshold score of 6 was identified. Using a revised threshold of 4, a sensitivity of 75% was observed. Specificity was not calculated because the *total sample* was composed of Mexican-American elders with affective disorder. There were no true negatives.

DISCUSSION

Although the different methodological approaches limit the capability to compare these populations, the results are presented because there have been few attempts to validate screening instruments for depression in populations of ethnic elders. With the changing demographic profile of the aging U.S. population, it will become increasingly important to know whether specific screening instruments may be used without modification in non-white populations. As emerging nations experience an improved economic base with resultant increased survival, the prevalence of affective illness in late life and affective illness associated with dementia can be expected to increase among non-white populations. Therefore, studies assessing the validity and reliability of screening instruments for affective disorder that can be administered by nonprofessional, trained interviewers have international implications for studies of non-white populations.

In the African American sample of community resident elderly, the GDS was only marginally effective as a screening instrument, providing a lower threshold of four was used. The psychiatric interview identified the presence of depressive symptoms which these black elders reported as symptoms of increased fatigue, a need to depend on their faith, and complaints of a worsening of chronic medical problem: "my sugar is up," "my blood pressure is bothering me more now," "I just have not felt well." Although a threshold of four will facilitate the identification of those African American elders with depressive symptoms, 36% of persons with depressive symptoms will be missed. In view of the studies that have used the CES-D in African American samples of mixed age, a study comparing the GDS, CES-D, and HDS would be a logical next step. If other samples of African American elders are found to report more somatic complaints and neurovegetative changes than guilty ruminations or suicidal ideation, screening instruments with these items would be preferable for these elders.

The results of the GDS-S among Mexican American elders with known affective disorder diagnosed by culturally-sensitive, psychiatrists familiar with the ethnic nuances suggest, again, that the screening test may have limited usefulness among Mexican American elders. The revised threshold improved the sensitivity to a minimally acceptable level of 78%. Due to the study design specific qualitative data on the specific complaints of these Mexican American elders on admission to the psychiatric unit was not obtained. Although the research assistant confirmed a pattern of somatic complaints of headache, stomach ache, muscle ache, and general feeling of fatigue in the sample, a detailed enumeration of symptoms on admission was not done. In view of our findings, a future study assessing the admission symptoms of patients rigorously diagnosed with affective disorder would be indicated. The use of multiple screening instruments which assess somatic and neurovegetative signs (Beck Depression Inventory & CES-D) in comparison to the GDS-S alone would provide important comparative data. The inclusion of a non-depressed sample of psychiatric patients would provide a subsample of true negatives and enable the calculation of specificity as well as sensitivity for this population.

These data were obtained from a clinical interview of African American elders. Although the nine, specific criteria for a DSM-III-R diagnosis of Major Depressive Disorder were explored, the majority of this sample of community-resident, African American elders did not report guilty ruminations, depressed mood, or problems with concentration. Their chief complaints involved worsening medical problems, the need to depend on their faith to help them through difficult times due to illness and conflict with neighbors, and the importance of a stoic attitude toward life. Both African American and Mexican American elders reported somatic complaints as depressive equivalents; joint pains, headache, gastrointestinal complaints, a general feeling of fatigue or a not being "up to par" or "well." Although level of acculturation for Mexican Americans has been reported to influence the report of psychiatric symptoms, the formal determination of place of birth and language of preference

(English or Spanish) was not done. Data from these studies do document that the African American and Mexican American elders in these samples did have a different pattern in the presentation of depressive illness.

The recent Consensus Conference on Depression in Late Life has emphasized the importance of carefully defining the severity of symptoms in order to include only patients with major depressive disorder (1992). The importance of adequate treatment with antidepressant medications was emphasized, also (National Institutes of Health, 1992). The importance of considering the difference in metabolism of psychopharmacologic agents was emphasized in a recent volume of psychopharmacology. Differences in the metabolism and distribution of psychoactive medications were discussed for African American (Strickland et al., 1991), Asian American, and Hispanic American populations (Mendoza et al., 1991).

CONCLUSION

The 15-item GDS was utilized to screen two populations of ethnic elders: community resident, African Americans and consecutively-admitted, Mexican Americans with affective disorders. In both samples the sensitivity was unacceptable using the original screening threshold of a score of six or more. Only with a revised threshold of four or more was the sensitivity improved to a minimally acceptable level of 75% among depressed, hospitalized, Mexican American elders. With the same adjustment of the threshold score, sensitivity among community resident African Americans was only 64%.

Future studies of populations of ethnic elders with rigorously diagnosed affective disorder are encouraged. In addition to the comparison of the GDS with instruments that include somatic and neurovegetative signs (CES-D, BDI, and the HDS) the importance of including a recording of the qualitative complaints of these depressed, ethnic elders is emphasized. Documentation of a difference in the presentation of depressive disorder among ethnic elders is needed. A broader knowledge of the specific complaints will facilitate the identification of characteristic presentations of affective illness and whether, and in what ways, they differ from the older white population.

REFERENCES

Alexopoulos GS, Young RC, Meyers BS. (1988). Late-onset depression. *Psychiatric Clinics of North America 11*:101-115.

Alexopoulos GS, Abrahams RC. (1991). Depression in Alzheimer's Disease. *Psychiatric Clinics of North America 14*:327-340.

Aneshensel CS, Clark VA, Frerichs RR. (1983). Race, ethnicity, and depression: a confirmatory analysis. *Journal of Personality and Social Psychology 44*(2): 385-398.

Angel JL, Hogan DP. (1991). The demography of minority aging populations. In *Minority Elders: Longevity, Economics, and Health. Building a Public Policy Base*, Harootyan LK (Ed). Washington, DC: The Gerontological Society of America, pp 1-13.

Baker FM, Lightfoot GB. (1993). Geriatric psychiatry, the evaluation and treatment of psychiatric disorders in ethnic elders. In Gaw AC (Ed). *Culture, Ethnicity, and Mental Illness*. Washington, DC: American Psychiatric Press.

Baker FM, Lavizza-Mourie R, Jorres BE. Acute care of the African American elder. *Journal of Geriatric Psychiatry and Neurology*. In Press.

Barón AE, Manson SM, Ackerman LM, Brenneman DL. Depressive symptomatology in older American Indians with chronic disease: some psychometric considerations (special report). Denver, CO: National Center for American Indian and Alaska Native Mental Health Research, University of Colorado Health Sciences Center.

Beck AT, Ward CH, Mendelson M. (1981). An inventory for measuring depression. *Archives of General Psychiatry 4*:53-63.

Blazer, D. (1988). Affective disorder in late life. In Busse EW & Blazer DG (Eds). *Geriatric Psychiatry*. Washington DC: American Psychiatric Press, pp. 369-401.

Brink TL. (Ed.) (1992). *Hispanic Aged Mental Health*. New York: The Haworth Press, Inc.

Burnam MA, Hough RI, Karno M, Escobar JI, Telles CA. (1987). Acculturation and lifetime prevalence of psychiatric disorders among Mexican Americans in Los Angeles. *Journal of Health and Social Behavior 28*:89-102.

Cassem NH. (1988). Depression secondary to medical illness. In Frances AS & Hales RE (Eds). *Review of Psychiatry Volume 7*. Washington, DC: American Psychiatric Press, pp 256-273.

Gurland BS. (1976). The comparative frequency of depression in various age groups. *Journal of Gerontology 31*:282-292.

Hamilton M. (1960). A rating scale for depression. *Journal of Neurology, Neurosurgery, and Psychiatry 23*:56-62.

Mendoza R, Smith MW, Poland RE, Lin KM, Strickland TL. (1991). Ethnic psychopharmacology: The Hispanic and Native American Perspective. *Psychopharmacology Bulletin 27* (4) :449-461.

Mezzich JE, Kleinman A, Fabregatt, Good B, Johnson-Powell G, Lin KM, Manson S, Parron D. (1992). Cultural Proposals for DSM-IV. Pittsburgh, PA: Western Psychiatric Institute.

Murrell S, Himmelfarb S, Wright K. (1986). Prevalence of depression and its correlates in older adults. *American Journal of Epidemiology 124*:372-388.

National Institutes on Health. (1992). *Concensus Development Conference on the Diagnosis and Treatment of Depression in Late Life*. Bethesda, MD: National Institutes of Health.

Neighbor HW, Jackson JS, Campbell L, Williams D. (1989). The influence of racial factors on psychiatric diagnosis: a review and suggestions for research. *Community Mental Health Journal 25*:301-311.

O'Connor DW, Pollitt PA, Roth M. (1990). Memory complaints and impairment in normal, depressed, and demented elderly persons identified in a community survey. *Archives of General Psychiatry 47*:224-227.

Powell GJ. (1982). Overview of the epidemiology of mental illness among Afro-Americans. In Bass BA, Wyatt GE, Powell GJ (Eds). Afro-American Family: Assessment, Treatment, and Research Issues, pp 155-163.

Roberts RE, Vernon SW, Rhoades HM. (1989). Effects of language and ethnic status on reliability and validity of the Center for Epidemiologic Studies–Depression Scale with psychiatric patients. *Journal of Nervous and Mental Disease 17*(10):581-592.

Rosenthal MP, Goldfarb NJ, Carlson BL, Sagi PC, Balaban DJ. (1987). Assessment of depression in a family practice center. *The Journal of Family Practice 25*:143-149.

Ruegg RG, Zisook S, Swerelow NR. (1988). Depression in the aged: an overview. *Psychiatric Clinics of North America 11*:83-99.

Sheikh JJ, Yesavage JA. (1986). Geriatric Depression Scale (GDS). Recent evidence and development of a shorter version. *Clinical Gerontologist 5*:165-173.

Sheikh JJ, Yesavage JA, Brooks JO. (1991). Proposed factor structure of the Geriatric Depression Scale. *International Psychogeriatrics 3*:23-28.

Smith-Ruiz D. (1985). Relationship between depression, social support, and physical illness among elderly blacks: research notes. *Journal of the National Medical Association 77*:1017-1019.

Strickland TL, Ranganath V, Lin KM, Poland RE, Mendoza R, Smith MW. (1991). Pharmacologic considerations in the treatment of black American populations. *Psychopharmacology Bulletin 27* (4) :441-448.

Vega WA, Kolody B, Warheit G. (1985). Psychoneuroses among Mexican Americans and other whites: prevalence and caseness. *American Journal of Public Health 75*:523-527.

Yesavage JA, Brink TL. (1983). Development and validation of a geriatric depression screening scale: a preliminary report. *Journal of Psychiatric Research 17*:37-49.

Sunk WWK. (1965). A self-rating depression scale. *Archives of General Psychiatry 12*:63-70.

SECTION TWO:
OUTREACH
TO THE FORGOTTEN

Chapter Three

Elderly Orphans with Alzheimer's Disease: Non-Traditional Support Systems

Barbara A. Soniat, MSW, PhD
Mona Pollack, MSW, PhD

Editor's Introduction

Soniat and Pollack shift our focus from assessment to out-reach. The "orphan elders" are those who do not have close family members who can serve as caregivers. These elders rely upon makeshift networks of neighbors and agencies, and even unlikely sources. The authors suggest that the people who compose these networks be brought into the process of assessment and management.

In the United States, it is estimated that there are 4 million victims of Alzheimer's disease. The risk for cognitive dysfunction shows a sharp increase with advancing age. Approximately 10% of

Barbara A. Soniat is Assistant Professor and Mona Pollack is Geriatric Social Worker, both affiliated with the Department of Health Care Sciences, Division for Aging Studies and Services, George Washington University, Washington, DC 20037.

[Haworth co-indexing entry note]: "Elderly Orphans with Alzheimer's Disease: Non-Traditional Support Systems." Soniat, Barbara A., and Mona Pollack. Co-published simultaneously in *Clinical Gerontologist* (The Haworth Press, Inc.) Vol. 14, No. 1, 1993, pp. 33-44; and: *The Forgotten Aged: Ethnic, Psychiatric, and Societal Minorities* (ed: T. L. Brink) The Haworth Press, Inc., 1993, pp. 33-44. Multiple copies of this article/chapter may be purchased from The Haworth Document Delivery Center. Call 1-800-3-HAWORTH (1-800-342-9678) between 9:00 - 5:00 (EST) and ask for DOCUMENT DELIVERY CENTER.

the population over 65 years of age live with the illness. Over the age of 85, 47% have a dementing illness. This older group is increasing more rapidly than other segments of the population because of declining birth and mortality rates, and increased life-extending medical care. In addition to an increase in the number of elderly individuals, the already existing older population is itself aging. The "old old" are the fastest growing segment of the population, and the group most vulnerable to a dementing illness.

Among the older population, dementia is a major cause of cognitive and functional loss. Alzheimer's disease, the most common form of dementing illness, is characterized by progressive impairment of attention and learning ability, severe loss of memory, problems with communication, motor functions, and impaired judgement. Persons with a dementing illness have difficulty handling ordinary activities of daily living. As the disease progresses there may be behavioral disturbances, such as wandering, repetitive vocalizations, angry outbursts and hallucinations.

Research has firmly documented that families are the major support for cognitively impaired older persons who are living in the community. Mace and Rabins (1990) have described the characteristic behavior problems that caregivers of persons with dementing illness must manage. Wandering, sleep disturbances, and repetitive behaviors are often present. Catastrophic reactions are another characteristic of a demented person. In addition, the person often has a fluctuating emotional state that ranges from apathy to anger. As the disease progresses, there are problems in motor functions and speech. Simple tasks may become too difficult for the impaired person. The caregiver may have to take over many routine chores, such as the individual's daily grooming. Safety of the demented person becomes a central issue in the caregiving relationship. Family often becomes the decision maker in most areas of functioning, including locus of care.

Although the majority of older persons have family that provide care, changes in these traditional support systems are expected as the result of a lower birth rate, increases in life expectancy, later marriages, and more women in the work force. This is occurring at the same time as the number of functionally impaired individuals living alone in the community without assistance of immediate kin is increasing (Worobey & Angel, 1990). It is apparent, however, that the progressive, and global nature of Alzheimer's disease necessitates that someone in addition to the victim be involved in decision making for safety issues, financial matters, health decisions and locus of care.

There is a gap in the literature on the support systems of persons with dementing illnesses who do not have close family members to provide care and support. At the present time, there are no data on older persons with dementia who live in the community without close family members who are available to provide ongoing assistance and support. We do know that 5% of the older population never married and have no children. Spouses and children are the customary caregivers for patients with dementia. Approximately 38% of the elderly are widowed, divorced or separated, and therefore do not have a spouse to function as caregiver. Twenty five percent do not have children. Within these groups of older people, one is likely to find "elderly orphans." There are older persons who do not have traditional family caregiving networks. Among "elderly orphans" one is likely to find that some suffer from Alzheimer's Disease or other dementing illnesses. Many live in the community for years, with the support of non-family informal support networks. Virtually nothing is known about the caregiving network of the Alzheimer victim without family and how these networks function to maintain and support victims of Alzheimer's Disease. This chapter attempts to focus attention on identifying the care providers for these victims as well as exploring the relationship of this support system with formal providers of care.

FORMS OF SUPPORT SYSTEMS

Gibson (1972) and Cantor (1979) have used the concepts of "functionality of kin" and "functional support" to distinguish between the mere presence of a support element and the available capacity and role of a support element in providing meaningful assistance. The few reported studies of older persons without family (Cihen & Rajkowski, 1982; Stoller & Earl, 1983; Johnson & Catalano, 1981) suggest that functional friends and neighbors networks act in a compensatory manner, assuming many of the functions of family when family members are absent from the social network, but these studies did not specifically focus on the cognitively impaired. Caring for a cognitively impaired older person has been shown to be more stressful than caring for the older person with physical disabilities.

There is a lack of research efforts concerning the critical role of support networks of the "elderly orphan." Two major reasons account for neglect in research in this area. First, it is difficult to locate and to interview this population, and second the focus of social scientists has been on the family's abilities to cope with the demands of care. Yet, there is a population of between 1 and 2% of the elderly with cognitive impairments, that depends on non-family members to assist them with daily tasks and long range decisions.

Greene and Soniat (1991) distinguish a "functional family system" from an informal network that provides assistance. A functional system is characterized by both affectional and instrumental roles, as well as having long term involvement with the older person. The friends and neighbors who comprise an informal network, may be involved in a more circumscribed and transient manner. The following case vignette describes the role of a non-traditional informal support network in maintaining a cognitively impaired older person in the community.

Case Vignette: Informal Network

Miss H is an eighty-seven year old, never married, retired legal secretary. She has lived in her current neighborhood and apartment for the past fifty years. She is well known to many of the shop keepers, merchants, and local community service professionals (i.e., policeman, fireman, postal employees, bank personnel, etc.) in the area. Miss H has no known family. She and an older sister moved from the Mid-West as young adults. None of her neighbors are aware of any out of town kin. She has a will that leaves her rather modest estate to her church.

Miss H ambulates very slowly, but manages to get around well in her neighborhood, which is located near an urban downtown area. She stays close to home, especially since an incident two years ago when she became confused and disoriented while riding a public bus, and was unable to find her way back home. The police were contacted, knew her, and were able to transport her home.

Firemen from a station near her home regularly help her cross a busy intersection; assist her with packages, and check on her if they don't see her making her usual rounds through the neighborhood each day. The local grocery store that she frequents allows one of its baggers to deliver her purchases. The resident manager of her apartment building reminds her to pay her rent and utility bills, and makes sure that she neither forgets to pay them nor overpays. She is very well known to the manager and tellers at her bank; having retired from another branch of the same bank. The bank's manager helped her to arrange direct deposit of her social security and pension checks. She has a trust account at the bank that helps her to manage her investment income. An attorney who works for the bank does her income taxes each year. She also receives help from the bank's staff with check writing and balancing her checkbooks.

Miss H eats all of her meals at a nearby restaurant. She is well known to the staff there, who call her and offer to deliver meals to her apartment when she fails to show up, especially during inclement weather. She has her hair done periodically at a local beauty shop, but is otherwise disheveled and often wears dirty clothes. She refused to allow anyone inside her apartment, although several neighbors offered to help her with laundry and cleaning.

Miss H came to the attention of the health care system after a fall outside her apartment building. Her physical injuries were minor; however the emergency room physician was concerned because she was confused, disoriented and unable to name a next of kin.

She was admitted to the hospital for assessment of changed mental status, and referred to the social work department for discharge planning assistance. Miss H had not seen a physician since her regular doctor died ten years earlier. She was in good physical health, but found to have previously undiagnosed visual problems and dementia, probably of the Alzheimer's type. The hospital attending physician recommended nursing home placement. A guardian was also recommended, since Miss H refused voluntary nursing home placement. A conservator was recommended for management of finances.

The hospital received many inquires about Miss H's condition. Several of her neighbors visited, but were uncomfortable with her pleas to "get her out." She eventually agreed to give a durable power of attorney to the lawyer who did her taxes. Her minister was instrumental in convincing her to try, at least on a temporary basis, living in a retirement community that provided assisted living. During the transition from the hospital to the retirement community, her resident manager and minister saw the inside of her apartment, and were convinced that she could not return to living alone. Both agreed that if she returned home, she would never consent to having anyone help her with personal care and housekeeping on a regular basis. Miss H remained in the retirement community, but was able to avoid guardianship and conservatorship proceedings with the help from her informal support network.

Discussion

The above case illustrates that bank personnel, church members, shop keepers and others may function in narrowly defined roles that allow the person to stay in the community without coming to the attention of guardianship panels. However, the lack of long term involvement, and commitment beyond these narrowly defined roles leave tremendous concern regarding whether the older person receives appropriate services, and the needed protective arrangements. This is even more difficult when the older person has Alzheimer's disease. These networks are often composed of members who don't know each other, and therefore do not engage in efforts to coordinate and monitor caregiving. As Mace (1989) illustrates, cognitively impaired older persons vary in their functioning abilities from day to day and even from morning to evening. It is particularly frustrating for the caregiver since behavior has no rational basis. What often keeps the caregiver involved is the history of the relationship and the emotional ties to the person. When this history does not exist, caregiving relationships often end at the convenience of the support person. If no service providers have been involved to strengthen the older person's situation he may abruptly be placed in an institution, or have a guardian appointed who becomes responsible for making decisions.

As seen in the following case illustration, when functional family is involved, there are critical differences in how decisions are made and implemented.

Case Vignette: Functional Family System

Mr. H is an 87-year old bachelor with Alzheimer's Disease. He lives in a middle class neighborhood in the family home he has occupied since birth. Mr. H and his only sister cared for both their parents at home until their deaths. He continued to share the home with his sister, who also never married, until her death ten years ago. His only living relatives are two cousins who live out of state. They visit approximately every other month.

Mr. H is in relatively good health. His only physical health problems are gout and a history of skin cancer. He has a very poor memory and is confused about medical and other bills. He is independent with ADLs. He needs assistance with cooking and housecleaning, tasks he has never performed well.

In addition to his cousins, his support system consists of an elderly female neighbor who calls him daily, visits frequently, sets up medical appointments, provides transportation and accompanies him on medical visits. She also arranges and supervises home care workers. At the present time, home care services include one day a week maid service and Meals on Wheels. The Meals on Wheels volunteer has also become a friend, providing transportation to non-medical appointments and visiting on a weekly basis. A male neighbor visits sometimes, and is also available to drive him places he needs to go.

Mr. H was referred to a case management program after a fall in his home. He was on the floor for almost twenty-four hours, unable to summon help. His female neighbor, who generally called him daily, was on vacation at the time. Upon her return, she became very concerned about the level of responsibility she had assumed for Mr. H, and the fact that his safety seemed very dependent on her availability and involvement. She felt guilt about not having made other arrangements for him before going on vacation, and thought that perhaps it was time for Mr. H to consider nursing home placement, since he had no close family members who were available to assume responsibility for his care.

Discussion

For years, Mr. H's neighbors and distant kin compensated for his lack of close relatives to function in a caregiving role. However, this network functioned without clear, socially defined norms regarding role requirements, limits on responsibility and obligations. With professional intervention, Mr. H and his network members were able to define these limits and to accept help in arranging for additional formal services to supplement those provided by his network.

Mr. H agreed to allow his cousins to assist him with finances. Formal services were arranged to supplement them in this role through a bill paying program and assistance with taxes.

Mr. H's neighbor was willing to continue helping him with medical visits and checking on him, but felt uncomfortable about being responsible for emergencies. All agreed that an emergency response system, a daily telephone reassurance volunteer, and continuing daily visits from the Meals on Wheels volunteer would complement the neighbor's efforts. Mr. H was admitted to a case management program. A case manager was assigned to assume responsibility for ongoing assessment, service coordination and monitoring. The case manager arranged for Mr. H and his neighbor to visit an Adult Day Care Center, a Group Home, a Retirement Community and a Nursing Home. Although Mr. H is managing well at home with the extra assistance, everyone is aware of the progressive nature of his illness and the probability that he will need more care in the future.

In both case vignettes, the informal support network assumed roles and functions that are normally performed by close family members. These nontraditional support networks had the same needs for information, support and assistance that family caregivers require. Caregiver stress can be exacerbated within non-traditional support networks because of ambivalence about the appropriateness of assuming a caregiving role. As with traditional family support networks, a caregiving crisis often brings these networks to the attention of formal service providers. Without the assistance of the non-family informal system, older persons without close family caregivers and many with geographically distant kin, could not safely reside in the community during even the earlier stages of Alzheimer's Disease.

PRACTICE IMPLICATIONS

Professionals need to be aware that the older person with a dementing illness and no family often has a significant support network that needs to be included in the assessment process. Engaging these significant others is difficult. It may be possible to identify different ways to strengthen the existing system and in so doing support the older person in the community. During the assessment process different pieces of information may need to be collected. This may entail getting permission from the older person, and collecting information from collateral contacts. Neighbors may be more reliable informants than the Alzheimer patient in determining issues of exploitation and safety.

An important task for a provider of service is to engage the client and client's system in the assessment process. It is very difficult to achieve this first step when the older person's memory and behavior is unpredictable, and informal caregivers are not easily identified. In fact both the older person and the caregiver may not readily identify this role.

Services that help the Alzheimer patient remain in the community are often predicated on there being a family caregiver. For example, some personal care and homemaker respite services require an at home caregiver. Day care, which provides a structured safe environment for many hours of the day, usually requires that the Alzheimer victim be groomed and ready for transportation at a designated time. Without a caregiver in the home this is usually not possible.

The implications for the caregiver who is not a close family member may be to limit their assistance and rely more on formal services. This may put a particular burden on community based case management and adult protective services. Institutional placement, rather than alternative long-term care options may be decided prematurely. As with close family relationships, non-traditional caregivers will vary in the amount of time and the type of support they can provide. Close family often provides the daily hands-on care needed by the cognitively impaired, as well as emotional support. Cognitively impaired older persons use less formal services, with family members providing higher levels of care than other functionally disabled older persons (Birkel & Jones, 1989; Stoller & Pugliesi, 1988).

Often older persons with severe cognitive problems and no family become known to community-based case management programs, adult protective services, and emergency rooms. They command greater health and social service resources. Social workers involved with this population need to engage the informal helping network as quickly as possible. These contacts are vital in providing information critical in developing an intervention strategy, and are often the link in interpreting formal services to the cognitively impaired older person. An important goal of the service plan is to educate individuals in the helping network to the nature of cognitive impairments, and to the progressive course of dementing illness. Clarifying what the individual has been doing, and what they can reasonably do in the future, may help prevent burn-out. Provision of formal services and structuring the environment to maintain independence may enable the informal network to remain involved with the knowledge that there are professionals who will monitor the situation and step in, if needed. With key helpers identified, it may be possible for long-range planning to take place.

FUTURE STUDIES

Currently, there are a minimum of data of how older persons with dementing illnesses and no family caregiver meet everyday needs. Knowledge is also lacking about the resources that are available at critical times. Identification of the natural support network and use of professional services is essential in order to identify the unmet needs of this group, who, by the progressive nature of their illness, will be at risk for institutionalization. This information is crucial in developing linkages that will facilitate coordination, rather than duplication of the informal and formal support systems now being utilized by the community regarding a cognitively impaired older person with no family caregiver.

BIBLIOGRAPHY

Barer, B.M., MSW, & C.L. Johnson, PhD. (1990). A Critique of the Caregiving Literature. *The Gerontologist.* Vol. 30(1), 26-29.
Birkel, R.C., PhD, & C.J. Jones, MS. (1989). A Comparison of the Caregiving Networks of Dependent Elderly Individuals Who Are Lucid and Those Who Are Demented. *The Gerontologist.* Vol. 29(1), 114-119.

Cicirelli, V.G., PhD. (1981). Kin Relationships of Childless and One-Child Elderly In Relation To Social Services. *Journal of Gerontological Social Work*. Vol. 4(1), 19-33.

Coe, R.N., PhD, F.D. Wolinsky, PhD, D.K. Miller, MD, & J.M. Prendergast, MD. (1984). Complimentary and Compensatory Functions in Social Network Relationships Among the Elderly. *The Gerontologist*. Vol. 24(4), 396-400.

Cohen, C.I., MD, & J. Sokolovsky, PhD. (1979). Health-Seeking Behavior and Social Networks of the Aged Living in Single-Room Occupancy Hotels. *Journal of the American Geriatrics Society*. Vol. XXVII(6), 270-278.

Colerick, Elizabeth J.. PhD, & L.K. George, PhD. (1986). Predictors of Institutionalization Among Caregivers of Patients With Alzheimer's Disease. *Journal of the American Geriatric Society*. Vol. 34(7), 493-498.

Garland, Jeffery. (1985). Adaptation Skills in the Elderly, Their Supporters and Carers. *The British Journal of Psychology*. Vol. 58, 267-274.

George, Linda K., PhD, & L.P. Gwyther, ACSW. (1986). Caregiver Well-Being: A Multidimensional Examination of Family Caregivers of Demented Adults. *The Gerontologist*. Vol. 26(3), 253-259.

Goldberg, Gertrude S., R. Kantrow, E. Kremen, & L. Lauter. (1986). Spouseless, Childless, Elderly Women and Their Social Supports. *Social Work*. Vol. 31(2), 104-112.

Goodman, Catherine Chase, DSW. (1984). Natural Helping Among Older Adults. *The Gerontologist*. Vol. 24(2), 138-143.

Hays, Judith C., RN, MSN. (1986). Patient Symptoms and Family Coping. *Cancer Nursing*. Vol. 9(6), 317-325.

Johnson, C.L., PhD, & D.J. Catalano, MSW, MPH. (1981). Childless Elderly and their Family Supports. *The Gerontologist*. Vol. 21(6), 611-618.

Keith, Pat M., PhD. (1983). Patterns of Assistance among Parents and the Childless in Very Old Age: Implications for Practice. *Journal of Gerontological Social Work*. Vol. 6(1), 49-59.

Oktay, J.S., MSW, PhD, & P.J. Volland, MSW, MBA. (1987). Foster Home Care for the Frail Elderly as an Alternative to Nursing Home Care: An Experimental Evaluation. *American Journal of Public Health*. Vol. 77(12).

Ory, Marcia G., T.F. Williams, M. Emr, B. Lebolwitz, P. Rabins, J. Salloway, T. Sluss-Radbaugh, E. Wolff, & S. Zarit. (1985). Families, Informal Supports, and Alzheimer's Disease. *Research on Aging*. Vol. 7(4), 623-644.

Revicki, Dennis A. & J. Mitchell. (1986). Social Support Factor Structure in the Elderly. *Research on Aging*. Vol. 8(2), 232-238.

Rice, Susan, DSW. (1989). Single, Older Childless Women: Differences Between Never-Married and Widowed Women in Life Satisfaction and Social Support. *Journal of Gerontological Social Work*. Vol. 13(3/4), 35-47.

Rubinstein, Robert L., PhD. (1985). The Elderly Who Live Alone and Their Social Supports. *Annual Review of Gerontology*. Vol. 5, 165-193.

Sanier, Janet S., S. Ochs, & J.M. McGloin. (1979). Reaching and Serving the Mentally Frail Elderly. *Aging*. 293-294. 10-17.

Seltzer, Marsha Mailick. (1985). Informal Supports for the Aging Mentally Retarded Persons. *American Journal of Mental Deficiency.* Vol. 90(3), 259-265.

Smyer, Michael A., PhD. (1980). The Differential Usage of Services by Impaired Elderly. *Journal of Gerontology.* Vol. 35(2), 249-255.

Stoller, Elanor P., PhD & L.L. Earl, MEd. (1983). Help with Activities of Everyday Life: Sources of Support for the Noninstitutionalized Elderly. *The Gerontologist.* Vol. 83(1), 64-70.

Stoller, Elanor P. & K.L. Pugliesi. (1988). Informal Networks of Community-Based Elderly. *Research on Aging.* Vol. 10(4), 499-516.

Stull, Donald E. & A. Scarisbrick-Hauser. (1989). Never-Married Elderly: A Reassessment with Implications for Long-Term Care Policy. *Research on Aging.* Vol. 11(1), 124-139.

Tennstedt, Sharon L., PhD, J.B. McKinlay, PhD, & L.M. Sullivan, MA. (1989). Informal Care for Frail Elders: The Role of Secondary Caregivers. *The Gerontologist.* Vol. 29(5), 677-683.

Ward, Russell A., PhD. (1985). Informal Networks and Well-Being in Later Life: A Research Agenda. *The Gerontologist.* Vol. 25(1), 55-61.

Zarit, Steven H. & J.M. Zarit. (1982). Families Under Stress: Interventions for Caregivers of Senile Dementia Patients. *Psychotherapy: Theory, Research and Practice.* Vol. 19(4), 461-471.

Chapter Four

Therapeutic Issues
with Gay and Lesbian Elders

Graham J. McDougall, PhD, CS, RN

Editor's Introduction

McDougall helps sensitize us to issues of the homosexual aged, not only their stigmatized existence, but also their remarkable strengths and special needs.

Being old and being gay may seem like an overwhelming task to accomplish, since aging has its share of emotional challenges and

Graham J. McDougall is Assistant Professor-Gerontological Nursing, Frances Payne Bolton School of Nursing at Case Western Reserve University, Cleveland, OH. He is a Geriatric Nurse Practitioner and a Clinical Specialist in psychiatric and mental health nursing with dual ANA certifications. His ten year clinical practice is providing in-home mental health services to older adults and their families.

Address correspondence to: Graham J. McDougall, PhD, CS, RN, Assistant Professor-Gerontological Nursing, Frances Payne Bolton School of Nursing, 2121 Abington Road, Case Western Reserve University, Cleveland, OH 44106.

[Haworth co-indexing entry note]: "Therapeutic Issues with Gay and Lesbian Elders." McDougall, Graham J. Co-published simultaneously in *Clinical Gerontologist* (The Haworth Press, Inc.) Vol. 14, No. 1, 1993, pp. 45-57; and: *The Forgotten Aged: Ethnic, Psychiatric, and Societal Minorities* (ed: T. L. Brink) The Haworth Press, Inc., 1993, pp. 45-57. Multiple copies of this article/chapter may be purchased from The Haworth Document Delivery Center. Call 1-800-3-HAWORTH (1-800-342-9678) between 9:00 - 5:00 (EST) and ask for DOCUMENT DELIVERY CENTER.

45

concerns. Ten years ago Dawson (1982) estimated up to 3.5 million homosexual men and women, over the age of 60, were currently living in the United States. A more conservative estimate of 1.75 million was given by Berger in 1984. Loss is the predominant theme of aging in all older adults who experience many losses which often occur simultaneously, e.g., death of spouse and friends, retirement, change in social status and loss of status, loss of income or drastic reductions in income, decline in physical health, and impending death.

Emotional responses experienced by older people such as anxiety, depression, grief and mourning, guilt, helplessness, loneliness, are universal, which means that homosexuals as well as heterosexuals will experience similar emotions in old age. In general the mental health needs of the older homosexual are similar to the needs of the older heterosexual (Berger, 1984). There are differences, however, in the way both groups have learned to cope with the stresses of life (Berger, 1982).

To be old and gay demands adaptation that most people have never had to experience with life. Wolf (1982) conducted in-depth interviews with 100 older lesbians and gay men and documented their many strengths. These strengths include learning at an early age to fend for themselves; cultivating several noncareer interests; preserving friendships outside a lover relationship; increasing their personal autonomy; and adjusting easier to old age since homosexuality means one has to live with a stigmatized identity throughout life. As a result of these learned coping strategies, elderly homosexuals may be better prepared for old age and adjust easier to old age than elderly heterosexuals.

There is a paucity of published research on the mental health needs of the older gays and lesbians since many tend to be invisible. The goal of this chapter is to critically analyze the literature on the mental health of aging homosexual men and women from a developmental perspective. Myths, stereotypes, historical events, and developmental issues are evaluated in the context of stress and coping. Finally, the therapeutic issues discussed are anxiety, bereavement, homophobia, homosexual dissatisfaction, intimacy, and sexuality.

MYTHS AND STEREOTYPES
OF AGING AMONG HOMOSEXUALS

From 1977 to 1982 there were numerous references related to myths and stereotypes of aging homosexual men and women. Some of the myths perpetuated are: (1) Gay men experience accelerated aging and prefer younger men; (2) Gay men end up being lonely and alone in their old age; (3) Older gay men are depressed, sexually frustrated, and unhappy; (4) Aging in lesbians is less traumatic than for the gay male because she doesn't operate in the same highly physical setting of competitiveness; (5) Older lesbians are lonely, totally isolated, and without anyone to love or care about her in old age; and (6) Being gay causes problems in old age (Archbold, 1982; Berger, 1980, 1982; Friend, 1980; Kelly, 1977; Kimmel, 1978, 1979; Laner, 1978; Laner, 1979; Martin and Lyon, 1979; Morin and Garfinkle, 1978; and Raphael and Robinson, 1980).

Berger's (1980) exemplar study of 112 homosexual men, 40 years of age or older, found few of the negative stereotypes to be supported. The actual number of older individuals in this study was much smaller; 60-69 age group (n = 21) and the 70-79 age group (n = 12). Given the difficulty of recruiting 33 older gay men, Berger's sample was impressive. Factors that were identified and contributed to healthy psychological adaptation were integration into the gay community; commitment to homosexuality; low concern with concealment of sexual preference; and satisfactory sex life. These factors are valuable to a mental health professional who may be working with an older homosexual client. These correlates of health could be classified as coping strategies and would be helpful in assessing a client.

Gray and Dressel (1985) challenged previous findings on older gay males from a new perspective. The researchers used a sample consisting of 4,212 gay males who responded to a self-administered questionnaire in 1977. This is the largest sample of gay males available, 50 years and older throughout the United States and Canada, both in urban and rural settings. Various relationships were manipulated statistically using a control variable, the length of time engaged in homosexual activity. The researchers utilized a process of inductive logic, suggested from the data, to offer alternative interpretations and insight regarding the phenomenon of aging among gay males. Previous beliefs about the negative stereotypes associated with being old and gay have been attributed to the effects of aging in a youth oriented subculture. Suggestions, or alternative hypotheses, were offered to reconceptualize aging in older gay males, such as subculture opportunity, subcultural aging, subcultural socialization, and, cohort effect. The findings indicate that factors other than aging per se may be important in understanding the experiences of older gay men. Major criticisms of this study were the non-probability nature of the sample recruited and data from a 1977 research study.

Laner's (1979) investigation of "Personals" placed by heterosexual (n = 229) and homosexual (n = 273) women to determine if older women of both sexual orientations would be overrepresented produced curious findings. Lesbians may have an advantage over nonlesbians since far fewer lesbians claimed their own age and concomitantly restricted the age of the prospective ad respondent. There was also no affirmation to support the belief that homosexual women are potential seductresses of the young. In a qualitative study, Raphael and Robinson (1980) investigated attitudes toward and preparation for aging, kinship/friendship networks, friends and lovers, identity and community in 20 self-identified lesbian women over the age of 50. Thanks to the excellent works of these investigators, the body of knowledge pertaining to aging homosexuals has increased; however, it does not identify the diversity in adult development among these individuals. This cohort of adults, before 1960, had very different life experiences than the cohort past 1970.

Older homosexuals are quite different from their younger counterparts and have different values and beliefs based on their life's experiences and historical events such as, pre-Stonewall, Great Depression, and the McCarthy investigations. Older gays bring with them these historical factors. These individuals grew up during a time of concealment during the 1930's before the sexual revolution. The Gay Liberation movement did not occur until 1970. These men and women had to be secretive to survive, in fact gay bars did not even appear until after World War II. A primary difference between older gays and younger gays is the bar scene. Older gays do not frequent the bars; they tend to have more parties with private circles of friends.

THERAPEUTIC ISSUES OF OLDER GAYS AND LESBIANS

Kimmel (1977) interviewed a group of fourteen gay men who ranged in age from 55 to 81, with a median age of 63 and identified two major differences that will be of concern in the treatment of the older gay male, the variety of gay lifestyles and the effect of a repressive social environment on the older gay male. These two differences are mentioned because each presents the therapist with a range of possible treatment modalities. Kimmel advocates using the range of services available to the gay community and being creative with the types of therapy prescribed to older gay males.

Gay men will seek the services of a psychotherapist for a variety of reasons just as do all other individuals who are having problems coping with life and are experiencing emotional pain. Whatever the reason for the therapy, the psychotherapist's role is to promote and facilitate growth in the client. The therapist must be aware of personal values and attitudes when treating a homosexual client so as to not subtly disapprove of the homosexual lifestyle. Martin (1982) mentions that the views society has about homosexuals are a reflection of two realities: homosexuality is deeply stigmatized in our society and homosexuals are largely invisible to society, so that the stigmatization goes mostly unchallenged. There is probably disagreement with being "unnoticed" at this time due to the AIDS crisis. The common therapeutic issues of anxiety, bereavement, homophobia, homosexual dissatisfaction, intimacy, and sexuality issues will be addressed.

Anxiety. Older adults are at a strong risk of experiencing anxiety and stress related to illness and death. Both have been implicated in the disease processes of asthma, hypertension, and ulcers. Older gays and lesbians experience all the same stressors in life plus issues such as concealment of their sexuality, loss of support from family, and homophobia. Aging gay males are at a high risk for developing anxiety and this may manifest in the two forms, somatic and cognitive. Examples of cognitive manifestations of anxiety are rigid thinking to protectively exclude external stimuli; fear of being alone; and suspiciousness to the point of paranoid states. Cognitive expression of anxiety may produce depression, confusional states or incorrectly label a person as senile. The relationship between anxiety and health is an issue of increasing importance as society "grays." Since older people in general have a tendency to somatize their emotional problems, they will probably seek a medical doctor to gain relief from the physical manifestations of anxiety (Wan, 1983; Waxman, 1984).

Bereavement. All adults may have a difficult time dealing with the death of a spouse or a lover of many years. Pathological bereavement is not easily predictable; however, a combination of the previous factors may indicate when normal grief becomes unresolved or changes its form to a depression. Since many older adults have a chronic illness, depressive reactions are often associated with physical disease, and often take the form of physical complaints; therefore making a diagnosis complicated. Increased dependency needs resulting from physical illness are a central issue to be addressed when providing psychotherapy with older adults.

Kimmel (1977) believes that bereavement is one of the few issues for which an older gay male will seek counseling or psychotherapy. However, Siegal and Hoefer (1981) think gay survivors are so deeply depressed by the time they seek professional help that they are self-destructive and already engaged in increased drug and alcohol use, masochistic behavior, obsessive interludes during work, quickly taking a new lover after the spouse's death (regardless of differences in age and temperament); and give in to general aimlessness. Community support programs and self help groups are other means to offer assistance to older gays and lesbians, and are often only found in large urban settings. A model program is SAGE (Senior Action in a Gay Environment) in New York City which offers free services to older gay men and women. Prime Timers is an example of a self help group started in Boston by individuals and is available in other parts of the country. Kimmel (1978) recommends that community centers offer specific outreach programs to the gay and lesbian community for bereavement, physical disability, and stigmatization.

Homophobia. One of the greatest problems any gay person must deal with is "Homophobia." Homophobia can be defined from two perspectives, cultural and personal. From a cultural perspective, homophobia is as any belief system which supports negative myths and stereotypes about homosexual people. More specifically, it can be used to describe: (1) belief systems which hold that discrimination on the basis of sexual orientation is justifiable; (2) the use of language or slang, e.g., "queer," which is offensive to gay people; and/or (3) any system which does not value homosexual lifestyles equally with heterosexual lifestyles (Morin and Garfinkle, 1978). From a personal perspective, homophobia refers to an irrational fear, or intolerance of homosexuals and homosexuality (Lehne, 1976).

Why then does homophobia become the worst enemy of the older gays? Since homosexuals know at an early age that they are different from heterosexuals a type of self-hatred is often present. Since heterosexuals usually hold strong beliefs regarding the gender roles, then the gay and lesbian individuals may internalize society's rejection of the homosexual. Therefore, homophobia becomes a specific condition or "phobia" that an individual develops. Older gays must have an awareness of this internalized self-hatred based on other people's irrational fears.

Many gay people become stuck with these irrational fears which surface as self-destructive behaviors. These self-destructive issues need to be exposed in order for the client to move into more self-accepting behaviors. The therapist must be aware of the gay person using derogatory slangs or terms such as "queer," faggot, fruit or using feminine pronouns when referring to self or others. This may indicate an individual is not consciously aware of his internalized hatred of homosexuals.

Homosexual dissatisfaction. Not all homosexuals are satisfied with themselves and their sexuality. Schwartz and Masters (1984) have developed a short-term intensive intervention adapted from the Masters and Johnson model for treating heterosexual disorders to treat men who want to change their homosexual preference. The directive psychotherapy alternates between confrontation of maladaptive belief systems and patterns of relating and support for finding new ways of coping that foster a positive self-image. One part of the intervention consists of pretreatment counseling which aims at improving the patient's dating, sexual, and intimacy skills; creative problem solving; and stress management. Following the pretreatment period, the patient and opposite-sex partner live in social isolation and meet daily with a therapy team to address fears and anxieties about intimacy as they arise.

Intimacy. Intimacy is a need basic to all humans; however, the way intimacy needs are met becomes the therapeutic issue. Loneliness, an emotional concern affecting all older adults, compels people to behave in many different ways and gays become lonely just as all other people do. The way loneliness is handled can be either positive or negative. There are many creative ways to handle issues of loneliness and meet intimacy needs among older persons, both gay and straight. Various styles of intimacy are described, neogamy being a generic term meaning new forms of intimate bonding and is described in this paper as those phenomena usually labeled alternative lifestyles (Dressel and Avant, 1978). Neogamy implies "new and therefore alternate forms of intimacy and bonding among individuals which may or may not be sexual." Neogamy is meant to replace the term "alternative lifestyles" which has pejorative connotations and implies deviance. Gay and lesbian individuals practice "neogamy" and the term is also appropriate to describe creative relationships of older persons in general. The types of neogamous relationships that will be discussed are cohabitation, polygyny, and communal arrangements.

Cohabitation is a coping strategy many older and unmarried people use to maintain maximum Social Security benefits, widow's pensions, intimacy and/or to eliminate children's worries of losing their inheritance, thereby diminishing their possible interference with the relationship. The author quotes statistics from 1970 and 1977 showing that the number of unmarried elderly couples of the opposite sex living together has increased from 18,000 to 85,000. While part of this figure represents landlord-tenant or head of household-paid employee relationships, the likelihood is that a substantial portion of these unmarried couples live as partners, since their ages tend to be similar. Cohabitation becomes an "unmarriage of convenience" for any number of reasons: sharing chores and expenses; meeting the needs of closeness and a sexual outlet; and alleviating loneliness.

Polygyny is another alternative living arrangement based on the imbalance in the same sex ratio among older people. Kassel (1966) discussed some of the social and emotional advantages of this lifestyle such as, obtaining group health insurance policies; division of household chores and care for the sick; improved diets and housing; creation of a family network; sexual outlet; and improving grooming. Polygyny is hypothetically a structural alternative addressing an imbalanced sex ratio; however, it seems unlikely that it will be legalized in the foreseeable future.

Communal arrangements may be useful for older people who do not mind sharing housing. Maggie Kuhn of the Grey Panthers advocates communal living arrangements of intergenerations. This intergenerational approach more appropriately resembles a nuclear family. In this arrangement, residents share economic resources and provide each other companionship and emotional support.

Homosexuality has also been considered as a means for older females to address unmet intimacy needs. This is based on the disproportionate number of older females to males.

Neogamy as an alternative method of meeting intimacy needs has many social prejudices to hurdle before being accepted. Legal obstacles, societal prejudice, and going against traditional family mores are some of the negative implications involved in acceptance.

How does neogamy apply to homosexual elders? Many gays grow into adulthood without role models and rarely does a young homosexual have meaningful contact with elderly gay and lesbian people. Most older homosexuals do not socialize in the bars and tend to entertain at home with close friends. This lack of a role model helps perpetuate some of the myths of aging among gays and aging in general. Since older people including older gays do have the special characteristics of wishing to leave a legacy, the elder function, and a sense of the entire life cycle, then younger gays might learn a great deal from having older role models (Butler and Lewis, 1982). Developing alternate forms of sharing intimacy is one way to perpetuate positive role modeling.

A community center or a social group may be an option for developing alternate forms of intimacy among gay males and lesbians, young and old. Castleman (1981) identified that a significant problem for older gays was a scarcity of social service programs that attend to the needs of older homosexuals. A center offering programs to all ages and sexes of gays and lesbians would allow for socialization. Younger gays then will have exposure to older gays and through interaction learn some of the coping strategies used by the older gays; also, some of the alternative living arrangements such as cohabitation, renting of rooms to college students, and other combinations of the above.

Sexuality. Sexuality and aging is another area where little research has been done. There are many myths about older adults and sexuality, i.e., (1) older people are dirty if interested in sex; (2) they can't make love anyway; (3) sexuality is lost with advancing age; and (4) physically unattractive people are not sexually desirable. Older men become the object of jokes such as being called "dirty old men." Fear about loss of sexual prowess is a common preoccupation for the older man and can reach devastating proportions (Butler and Lewis, 1982).

In a study that analyses attitude changes within five cohorts about sexual morality, Cutler (1985) found no evidence of a conservative shift in attitudes. Data were taken from nine nationally representative surveys of the adult population in the U.S. over the period 1972-1982. Three topics were used to measure attitudes about sexual morality because it taps a central facet of the liberal/conservative dimension which is labelled as "permissiveness": premarital sexual relations; extramarital sexual relations; and homosexual relations. There were no significant differences in change of attitudes between older and younger cohorts over the time period. The findings disclosed a consistent conservative pattern across the three items.

Merrie (1981) describes a process leading to decreased sexual expression in the elderly people as the "Geriatric Sexuality Breakdown Syndrome." This syndrome occurs in seven steps. Step one occurs with physiological changes in the sexual response cycle that occur with aging. Also, sociological changes in loss of role may diminish sexual expression. Step two is characterized by increased dependence on cues from society which are usually negative. Step three is labeling such as "dirty old man" or "indecent old woman." This labeling affects general well-being by decreasing self-esteem.

Step four is the adoption of the sick role by the elderly. Step five is the learning of behaviors and skills appropriate to the sick role. Step six is characterized by an atrophy of work and social skills. At this step the elderly persons may begin to see themselves as asexual or neuter. Step seven occurs when masculine or feminine identification is threatened. This step is finalized with the incorporation of the terms "dirty old man" and "indecent old woman."

Sex education may be important in preventing this cycle from occurring. Since the elderly grew up around the turn of the century, it is doubtful that factual information about sexuality and aging is known to them. One study was conducted to assess the effects of an older age oriented sex education program on elderly persons, nursing home staff, and adult family members of elderly persons (White and Catania, 1982). Sexual intercourse was increased by 400% as a consequence of this program.

In one study of older gay males, sex role flexibility described as not adhering to a strict masculine sex role correlated positively with aging (Friend, 1980). Gay males have the advantage of being flexible in their sexual roles if they do not adhere to a strict masculine sex role. This flexibility challenges stereotyped roles for males. A therapist who can validate a gay male's creative violation of sex role stereotypes and use this issue therapeutically is wise. Heterosexual men may learn a great deal from the mixture of roles gay men experience in their relationships.

CONCLUSION

This paper evaluated the mental health concerns of older gays and lesbians as identified in the literature. Many of the myths concerning older homosexuals have been dispelled through research. The therapeutic issues affecting this cohort of older adults are: anxiety, bereavement, homophobia, homosexual dissatisfaction, intimacy, and sexuality. Older homosexuals have strengths and weaknesses just as all other people; however, they have additional coping strategies which allow them to enter old age at an advantage. The task of the therapist treating an older homosexual client is to support and strengthen effective coping strategies and discard ineffective ones.

REFERENCES

Archbold, R. (1982). Growing old, staying young. *The Body Politic*, December, 25-28.

Berger, R. M. (1980). Psychological adaptation of the older homosexual male. *Journal of Homosexuality, 5*(3), 161-175.

Berger, R. M. (1982). *Gay and Gray*. Chicago, IL: University of Illinois Press.

Berger, R. M. (1982). The unseen minority: Older gays and lesbians. *Social Work*, May, 236-242.

Berger, R. M. (1984). Realities of gay and lesbian aging. *Social Work*, Jan-Feb, 57-62.

Butler, R. N. & Lewis, M. I. (1982). *Aging and mental health* (3rd ed.). St. Louis, MO: C. V. Mosby.

Castleman, M. (1981). Growing older homosexual. *Medical Self Care, 15*, Winter, 20.

Cutler, S. J. (1985). Ageing and attitudes about sexual morality. *Ageing and Society, 5*, 161-173.

Dressel, P. L. & Avant, W. R. (1978). Neogamy and older persons. *Alternative Lifestyles, 1*(1), 13-37.

Friend, R. A. (1980). Gaying: Adjustment and the older gay male. *Alternative Lifestyles, 3*(2), 231-248.

Gray, H. & Dressel, P. (1985). Alternative interpretations of aging among gay males. *The Gerontologist, 25*(1), 83-87.

Kassel, V. (1966). Polygyny after 60. *Geriatrics, 21*(4), 214-218.

Kelly, J. (1977). The aging male homosexual myth and reality. *The Gerontologist, 17*(4), 328-332.

Kimmel, D. C. (1977). Psychotherapy and the older gay man. *Psychotherapy: Theory, Research and Practice, 14*(4), 386-393.

Kimmel, D. C. (1978). Adult development and aging: A gay perspective. *Journal of Social Issues, 34*(3), 113-130.

Kimmel, D. C. (1979). Adjustments to aging among gay men. In B. Bergon & R. Leighton (Eds.), *Positively Gay* (pp. 146-158). California: Celestial Arts.

Kimmel, D. C. (1979-80). Life-history interviews of aging gay men. *International Journal of Aging and Human Development, 10*(3), 239-248.

Laner, M. R. (1978). Growing older male: Heterosexual and homosexual. *The Gerontologist, 18*(5), 496-501.

Laner, M. R. (1979). Growing older female: Heterosexual and homosexual. *Journal of Homosexuality, 4*(3), 267-275.

Lehne, G. K. (1976). Homophobia among men. In D. David & R. Brannon (Eds.), *The forty nine percent majority: The male sex role*. New York: Addison-Wesley.

Martin, A. (1982). Some issues in the treatment of gay and lesbian patients. *Psychotherapy: Theory, Research and Practice, 19*(3), 341-348.

Martin, A. & Lyon, P. (1979). The older lesbian. In B. Bergon & R. Leighton (Eds.), *Positively Gay*. Millbrae, CA: Celestial Arts.

Merrie, J. K. (1981). Geriatric sexuality breakdown syndrome. *International Journal of Aging and Human Development, 13*(1), 71-77.

Morrin, S. F. & Garfinkle, E. M. (1978). Male homophobia. *Journal of Social Issues, 11*(1), 29-47.

Raphael, S. M. & Robinson, M. K. (1980). The older lesbian. *Alternative Lifestyles, 3*(2), 207-229.

Schwartz, M. E. & Masters, W. H. (1984). The Masters and Johnson treatment program for dissatisfied homosexual men. *American Journal of Psychiatry, 141*(2), 173-181.

Siegel, R. L. & Hoefer, D. D. (1981). Bereavement counseling for gay men. *American Journal of Psychotherapy, 35*(4), 517-525.

Wan, T. T. H. & Arling, G. (1983). Differential use of health services among the disabled elderly. *Research on Aging, 5*(3), 411-431.

Waxman, H. M., Carner, E. A. & Klein, M. A. (1984). Underutilization of mental health professionals by community elderly. *The Gerontologist, 24*(1), 23-30.

White, C. B. & Catania, J. A. (1982). Psychoeducational intervention for sexuality with the aged, family members of the aged and people who work with the aged. *International Journal of Aging and Human Development, 15*(2), 121-138.

Wolf, D. G. (1982). *Growing Older: Lesbians and Gay Men.* California: University of California Press.

Chapter Five

Practice with Older Parents
of Developmentally Disabled Adults

Gregory C. Smith, EdD
Sheldon S. Tobin, PhD

Editor's Introduction

Smith and Tobin look at aged parents who are still stuck in the role of caregivers to their own children, adult offspring with developmental disabilities. The authors focus on the family context and outreach is blended with some counter-transference issues which therapists and case workers may experience in working with this population.

Gregory C. Smith is affiliated with the Department of Human Development, University of Maryland, College Park, MD 20742. Sheldon S. Tobin is affiliated with the Ringel Institute of Gerontology, University at Albany-SUNY, Albany, NY 12222.

This study was funded by NIA Grant #RO1 AG09198, Permanent Residential Planning By Parents of MR Adults and, in part, by support to the first author from the General Research Board of the University of Maryland, College Park.

[Haworth co-indexing entry note]: "Practice with Older Parents of Developmentally Disabled Adults." Smith, Gregory C., and Sheldon S. Tobin. Co-published simultaneously in *Clinical Gerontologist* (The Haworth Press, Inc.) Vol. 14, No. 1, 1993, pp. 59-77; and: *The Forgotten Aged: Ethnic, Psychiatric, and Societal Minorities* (ed: T. L. Brink) The Haworth Press, Inc., 1993, pp. 59-77. Multiple copies of this article/chapter may be purchased from The Haworth Document Delivery Center. Call 1-800-3-HAWORTH (1-800-342-9678) between 9:00 - 5:00 (EST) and ask for DOCUMENT DELIVERY CENTER.

Gerontologists have become increasingly concerned and knowledgeable about issues that confront family caregivers to the frail elderly. Indeed, despite the great diversity that exists among this caregiver population, providing care to an elderly family member is often regarded as a normative life task (Brody, 1985). Overlooked by gerontologists, however, has been an expanding population of family caregivers whose situation is strikingly non-normative in nature, namely older parents of developmentally disabled adults.

Described in this chapter is the manner in which both the developmental and caregiving circumstances of these parents is non-normative, and then significant concepts related to practice with this target population are elucidated. Three sources have informed us regarding the issues discussed in this chapter: a study of 235 mothers, age 58 to 96, who provide care at home to a son or daughter with mental retardation; in-depth interviews with 11 experienced case managers who serve these families, and discussions with various other clinicians and administrators from both the aging and developmental disability service networks. First, however, it is necessary to define being a caregiver to a developmentally disabled offspring.

According to Public Law 95-602, a developmental disability is a severe and chronic disability that is attributable to a mental or physical impairment, manifests before age 22, is likely to continue indefinitely, results in substantial functional limitations in three or more areas of major life activity, and reflects the need for a combination and sequence of special individualized services that are lifelong or of an extended duration (Lippman & Loberg, 1985). Typically, developmentally disabled persons have one or more of the following conditions: mental retardation, cerebral palsy, autism, sensory impairments, neurological impairments, and various other lifelong disabilities.

Obviously, then, there is considerable diversity among the population of developmentally disabled adults that must be reflected in programs and services for these individuals and their families. Nevertheless, because the overwhelming majority of developmentally disabled persons surviving to later adulthood are mentally retarded (Lubin & Kiely, 1985), more knowledge is available about these

families than for those confronted by other developmental disabilities.

Gerontologists have heretofore passed over the concerns of parents of developmentally disabled adults because, until recently, parental caregiving ended prior to old age as offspring succumbed during early stages of the family life cycle. As a result, however, of such influences as deinstitutionalization, decreased mortality rates, improved health care, the aging of the baby boom generation, and expanded community services, there has been an accelerated increase in the numbers of families in which elderly parents function as caregivers to a developmentally disabled son or daughter (Janicki & Wisniewski, 1985). Thus, professionals from the fields of both gerontology and developmental disabilities are now faced with the task of addressing the service needs of these families (Sison & Cotten, 1989; G. C. Smith & Tobin, 1989).

NON-NORMATIVE PARENTAL CAREGIVING

Effective practice with older parents of developmentally disabled adults must be informed by knowledge of how both their psychological developmental and caregiving arrangements are uniquely different from those of most older persons. Normative aging can be characterized as having no "unfinished business," at the end of the life course (Tobin, 1991). The self, one's personhood, is preserved by lessening expectations of what can be controlled but being able to do and control some things that are personally meaningful; by blending the past with the present in one's self picture; and dramatizing the past, to make oneself vivid to self. The past is also important for the maintenance of subjective well-being because of the importance of being able to perceive a congruence between expected and achieved life goals (Neugarten, Havighurst & Tobin, 1961). Death becomes acceptable as the concern shifts to the process of dying, to not wishing to die also, in unendurable pain, immobile and intractably confused. Making death, as well as age itself, acceptable to most Americans are their religious beliefs; that is, three of God's blessings: a long life (beyond the three score and ten that most people now exceed) as a divine reward for service, relief when in unendurable suffering, and reunions in the afterlife.

In normative aging, success in the rearing and launching of children among women enables the perception of a congruence between expected and achieved life goals and, also, past mothering provides evidence for the current self-picture. Caregiving first to parents and then later to husbands supports women's self-view of being nurturant and caring, and is a source of gratification when having onerous caregiving tasks to perform and becoming overwhelmed by caregiving burden.

In contrast, non-normative aging in the context of this paper refers to having life tasks uncompleted later in life. Parents of offspring with developmental disabilities are not the only ones encompassed in this definition. Witness active visual artists (Tobin, 1991): Hokasai, the greatest of Japanese woodcutters, who said on his deathbed at 94, "I am just beginning to learn my craft." Parents of developmentally disabled adults, of course, differ from active visual artists, but they also differ from parents caring for offspring with mental illness because usually the children of these latter parents did not manifest their illness in their earliest years (Lefly, 1987). For offspring with developmental disabilities, caring has been a lifelong task. They are "perpetual parents" (Jennings, 1987) who should make future plans for the time after their deaths that encompass financial, guardianship and especially permanent residential plans.

The problems that confront older parents in long-range planning are both logistically complex and emotionally draining. Known as "permanency planning," this effort requires resolution of the guilt and anxiety over relinquishing the care of one's dependent offspring, as well as the making of difficult decisions regarding financial security, guardianship, and residential placement (M. M. Seltzer & G. B. Seltzer, 1985; G. C. Smith & Tobin, 1989). Practitioners must assist parents with permanency planning not only to ease parents' uncertainties and insure smooth transitions for their mentally retarded offspring, but also to insure that the public sector will not be overwhelmed by a wave of new clientele who unexpectedly need publicly supported residences upon the death of older parents. Unfortunately, today's practitioners have not established guidelines to direct their efforts in providing permanency planning assistance.

Permanent residential plans, specifically relocation to a nursing home, may occur in caregiving to a frail elderly family member; that is, in normative parent-caring and normative spouse-caring. If the elderly care receiver is relocated to a nursing home, these caregivers, too, feel they are abandoning their loved ones (Tobin & Lieberman, 1976). These feelings may not be dissimilar to those felt by non-normative caregivers to disabled adults who anticipate a final separation. All caregivers who even contemplate relocation know only too well that no one can provide their kind of tender, loving care. Still, it differs for older mothers of developmentally disabled offspring not only because current caregiving is very gratifying but also because it is their own deaths, which weigh heavily on their minds, that will bring the final separation. Daughters and spouses after institutionalizing parents and spouses, and then after the deaths of these elderly family members, continue their lives usually feeling after awhile that they cared appropriately. They need not deny their aging or not be accepting of their deaths.

At another level, what most bothers family caregivers to elderly members, may reflect beneficial ways of adapting (Tobin, 1991). It is, for example, best for elderly care receivers to maintain persistent life long psychodynamics and interpersonal dyadic styles with their caregivers, but these psychodynamics and styles can indeed be disturbing, especially to children who can feel infantilized or inadequate. Most severe may be the daughter who took on caregiving to gain the love she feels was given to the favorite daughter, her sister; but unfavorable comparisons will still be made with her sister. Also good for the elderly care receiver is to reminiscence, but repetitious reminiscence can become odious. In turn, facilitatory over-inflated beliefs in mastery can be frightening. And expressions of aggressivity, which facilitate adaptation to stress in aging (Lieberman & Tobin, 1982; Tobin & Lieberman, 1976), can become constant irritations.

These sources of discomfort interact with feelings of inadequacy in caregiving to cause anger toward oneself but also augment the usually suppressed anger toward the care receiver for placing her in this position. The dynamics are quite different for perpetual parents. Sought, for example, is the stability of the psychodynamics in the relationship. Anger is not likely to be felt toward self or the offspring; rather it is generally externalized and directed toward those who stigmatize their child or providers who do not care enough.

Both normative and non-normative caregivers, however, have problems related to control. G. C. Smith, M. F. Smith and Toseland (1991), for example, found that daughter and daughter-in-law care givers in counseling introduced pressing problems largely related to control. Ambivalent feelings regarding control were produced by the wish to permit parents and parents-in-law as much autonomy as possible versus the need to care and protect them. Concurrently, lack of time for husbands but time-consuming caregiving reduced a sense of control of the situation. Time management was a critical issue for these caregivers who felt they were being controlled rather than being in control. Exacerbating dilemmas around control were feelings toward their siblings' involvement in caregiving. Many felt that rather than nag siblings to share more of the burden, it was best to cope with their anger and resentment by saying nothing and suppressing these emotions. Indeed, it was common to focus on what could be controlled but with underlying disturbing feelings that included anxiety about a caregiving situation that could easily go out of control. As one caregiver said, "I can't handle anything negative. I always try to ignore it." Compounding their inner-state was the realization that as another caregiver said, "I must understand that mom won't be there for me emotionally. I must meet that need myself." Then, they too, like the non-normative mothers, feared the future of their caregiving which focused on mothers' deterioration and nursing home placement.

Non-normative caregivers to their offspring with MR are different. From a lifetime of caring that is perceived as successful, they feel in control of everyday life. To be sure, disability-related decrements in their offspring and age-associated deterioration in themselves can cause difficulties. Our data, however, suggest that they cope well with these difficulties; and because of their ability to provide a home for their offspring, feel very much in control. Maybe, paradoxically, it is these very feelings of being very much in control in everyday life that make it even harder to accept the reality that they have no control over gross disabilities and their deaths.

DATA SOURCES

In all, 235 mothers, 58 to 95 years of age, were interviewed for two hours or so by experienced clinicians with masters degrees (Smith, Fullmer & Tobin, in press). Found was their paradoxical aging (Tobin, Fullmer & Smith, in press). As compared to normative aging mothers, they had greater subjective well-being but less acceptance of deaths with age. A high level of subjective well-being, evidenced on the Bradburn's (1969) Affect Scale (the BABS) and the Neugarten, Havighurst and Tobin (1961) Life Satisfaction Rating (LSR), was congruent with the high degree of current satisfactions in caregiving and also gratifications from rearing their offspring. With age, however, the confrontation with the necessity to make permanent residential plans for when they are gone causes an unwillingness to give in to their aging and to their deaths. Few could accept becoming old and, in contrast to normative aging, fears increased and acceptance of death lessened with age.

The resistance to making permanent residential plans was reflected in that nearly one-half had made no concrete plans, independent of age, which is consistent with the findings of others (Carswell & Hartig, 1979; Heller & Factor, 1991; Roberto, 1989; Wood & Skiles, 1992). Indeed, 47 (20%) of our 235 mothers, independent of age had not yet had any discussions of permanent residential plans. Related to not making plans in our sample of mothers was the purposive avoidance of any future planning; not accepting age-associated adverse changes in self; not having other children or having other children who are not providing much assistance to their parents or siblings with MR; and non-use or underutilization of available services for their offspring, as well as non-use of peer support groups. The use of support groups was not only associated with greater positive current effects on the BABS ($r = .19$) but also higher LSR (.27) and more acceptance of death (.19), as well as more permanent residential planning (.20). Also those mothers who used support groups were more educated (.22), had less ADL incapacity ($-.20$), used (.29) and had more knowledge of services (.24) for their offspring, and their offspring were younger ($-.18$).

Use of formal services is of particular importance because use of services apparently diminishes the perception that professionals intrude into their lives. Many of the oldest parents, however, have avoided services because when they birthed their offspring only institutional care was available and not services to assist in community care. Also the attitudes toward mental retardation were different. As one respondent said, "He (the doctor) said to throw him away like an old dish rag." Ironically, those who use services more are less satisfied with services. Our interviews suggest that these determined, strong-willed mothers who are very attuned to their offspring's needs are sensitive to any and all services they use that do not assist their offspring in meaningful ways.

The perceptions of case managers have been neglected. There are, however, exceptions depicting how case management should be modified when working with these parents (Sutton, Sterns, Schwartz & Roberts, 1992; Kaufman, DeWeaver & Glicken, 1989). Kaufman et al. (1989) discussed modifications in six roles of case management: outreach worker, advocate, teacher of parents, therapist, enabler/facilitator, and broker/coordinator. This theoretical discussion contrasts with our investigation of case managers' perceptions, a first such study, and also with our focus on permanency planning; that is, Kaufman et al., as well as Sutton et al., almost exclusively focused on maintaining family care at home.

The 11 case managers that we interviewed saw their assistance to parents with permanency planning issues as primarily involving two of the practice roles described by Kaufman et al. (1989). On the one hand, case managers must engage in the therapist role to help parents confront the emotion laden issues surrounding the anticipation of their own death and worry about what the future holds for their mentally retarded offspring. Simultaneously, the case manager must engage in the teacher role by clarifying for older parents what residential programs are available and how these programs are suited to the needs of their disabled offspring. Indeed, these two roles are interrelated to the extent that older parents will be better able to resolve their uncomfortable feelings regarding the future as they become increasingly aware that residential programs may not be as bad as they have assumed.

Our in-depth interviews with 11 case managers with lengthy experience in working with elderly parents revealed four themes: ageism is implicit in the MR/DD system, primarily because of the focus on quick outcomes; the system has some specific inadvertent deleterious aspects; older parents have greater needs for nurturance and emotional support; and case managers have frustrations, as well as thinly veiled anger, because of their perceptions that parents are selfish (Smith & Tobin, in press). The first theme, that there is ageism within the MR/DD service system is indicated by the case manager who said, "Ageism exists in the system. In this job, you're judged successful if you give services that result in outcome. So, the feeling is why work with older parents who will die. Your job tenure is threatened if you work too much with older parents." Also noted by the case managers was the system's emphasis on quick, positive outcomes that are less likely to be achieved with older families. If the rewards in the system are for efficiency, they said, then older families are likely to be compromised. The existence of ageism was further suggested by the failure to recognize heterogeneity among older parents. Indeed, only one case manager indicated that personality was more important than age in understanding older parents.

The second theme concerned aspects of the MR/DD system that are inadvertently deleterious to aging families. The case managers were discouraged, for example, by the paucity of available residential options, and noted that this exacerbates parents' avoidance of permanency planning. They also commented on how older mothers often worry about being seen as inadequate by the younger, better educated, and physically stronger women who comprise the majority of MR/DD professionals. This, they said, produces conflict and mistrust between parents and professionals. They noted further that the bureaucratic red tape of the MR/DD system is bewildering to many older parents who lack the stamina or patience to deal with it.

The third theme was that older families have special needs. As one case manager said, "Individual services don't work unless the older parent has someone to nurture them . . . The worker who sits down and drinks coffee with the parent is saying 'You're still valuable.' You just can't go in once a month to see that everything is ok. You must talk about more than just the child, even though this isn't seen by supervisors as your job . . . Working with older parents is a true social work task and we'd rather be doing this than a lot of paperwork."

It is the fourth theme, of frustrations and veiled anger, that especially reflects the articulation of mothers' attitudes toward practitioners and practitioners' attitudes towards parents. Mothers do not want to sever a lifetime of gratifying caregiving by making permanent residential plans for the time after their deaths. Practitioners, in turn, are conscious of the plight of these parents and how they must work gently and slowly with them. They also see the avoidance of making plans as somewhat selfish; that is, as comfortable for parents but with the possibility that on a late Friday afternoon, the offspring will be dumped on their door with no place to live and will have to be placed inappropriately either in an institution or a group home. One of the case managers reported, "A mother age 80 said that she'd kill her 47-year old daughter before placing her. And, this isn't uncommon!"

Discussions with other case managers, as well as administrators, in the MR/DD system and with personnel in the area agency network add further to understanding resistances by mothers to planning and by case managers to counseling parents and also to understanding the anger generated. Blame is indeed ubiquitous. Administrators blame case managers for not working enough with these parents while underplaying the pressures for quick results with large caseloads. Case managers blame administrators for not giving them the added time to work with these parents and also the needed residential resources. Area agency personnel blame both administrators and practitioners in the MR/DD system for ignoring these families. Then, the professionals in the MR/DD system dismiss the personnel in the area agency network for believing they can somehow, rather magically, assist these families in making permanent residential plans. Yet, there is a consensus that with the ever increasing numbers of these families, there is an urgent need to attend to the necessity of making permanent residential plans.

THE CONTEXT OF PRACTICE

Issues regarding practice will be discussed within three levels: the context of practice, outreach or the making of clients, and counseling to families. As shown in Chart 1, three initiatives have been identified to enhance the context of practice.

CHART 1. SOME ESSENTIAL PRACTICES WITH OLDER PARENTS

CONTEXT OF PRACTICE

> NEED FOR POLICIES THAT SUPPORT PRACTICE WITH AGING FAMILIES.
>
> EDUCATION AND TRAINING OF STAFF, ESPECIALLY CLINICIANS TO WORK WITH THESE FAMILIES.
> CONSIDERATION TO HAVING GERIATRIC SPECIALISTS.

OUTREACH TO MAKE PARENTS INTO CLIENTS

> EDUCATIONAL PROGRAMS SPONSORED UNDER NON-THREATENING AUSPICES.
>
> DEVELOPING AND NURTURING PEER SUPPORT GROUPS.
>
> SENIOR CENTER AND AREA AGENCY PERSONNEL SEEKING OUT PARENTS OF THEIR MR PARTICIPANTS TO RECRUIT THEM AS MR/DD CLIENTS.
>
> OUTREACH BY MR/DD STAFF.

COUNSELING

> GOING SLOWLY.
>
> APPRECIATING THE PLIGHT OF PARENTS REGARDING RESISTING AGING AND FEARS OF DEATH FROM THE NEED TO MAKE PERMANENT RESIDENTIAL PLANS.
>
> DIMINISHING FRUSTRATION AND ANGER.
>
> INCORPORATING OTHER CHILDREN, SIBLINGS OF THE OFFSPRING WITH MR, INTO COUNSELING ON PERMANENCY PLANNING.

Policies must change. Although increased attention has been given to interventions involving older individuals with retardation, interventions with aging families have been virtually ignored in the literature which apparently reflects a tendency in the MR/DD system to regard family members as merely resources for the disabled client, rather than recognizing that the family itself has needs (Slater & Wikler, 1986). This is evident in the proposed 1992-1993 legislative and social goals of the American Association on Mental Retardation which invoke the integration of elderly persons with mental retardation into mainstream aging services but fail to address the concerns of family caregivers. Moreover, without available living alternatives, especially group homes in adequate supply, effective permanency plans cannot be made.

Because the MR/DD system has been inattentive to these families, education and training is needed at many levels, especially for clinicians. The experienced clinicians we interviewed reported so many frustrations that they recommended more gerontological education and training specifically focused on counseling these aging parents.

Because of their own lack of knowledge and training, several of the case managers recommended that geriatric specialists be employed to work only with these families. An additional reason for this suggestion was the time-consuming nature of the counseling that also necessitates lower case loads. Also, geriatric specialists would be able to know how best to link parents who are failing in health to appropriate service providers and to the aging network.

OUTREACH TO MAKE PARENTS INTO CLIENTS

The difficulties in recruiting our sample of 235 women led us to learn about outreach programs. There have been at least two very successful outreach programs to those who have been characterized as "the hidden" because they are relatively unknown to the formal MR/DD service system (Home, 1989). A service-oriented project sponsored by the Rehabilitation Research and Training Center (RRTC) Consortium on Aging and Developmental Disabilities in Akron, Ohio, presented workshops on permanency planning that attracted many older parents of adults with mental retardation who were previously unknown to service providers. The workshops were advertised in newsletters associated with aging network programs, and were conducted under the auspices of a generic social service agency, the Jewish Community Center, rather than a provider from the mental retardation service system. Thus, parents' apprehension of mental retardation professionals was deliberately circumvented. Another effort to locate older underserved families was carried out in a five county area in rural Virginia by the Rappahannock-Rapidan Community Service Board, an organization that combines aging, mental health, developmental disability, and substance abuse agencies under one administrative umbrella (Rappahannock-Rapidan Community Services Board, unpublished manuscript). Apparently, this program, according to G. C. Smith, Fullmer and Tobin (in press), was productive for three reasons: first, it was funded by a federal grant which supported a full-time outreach worker. Second, professionals from the aging agency could be easily reached and trained to identify and refer aging families because their agency was under the administrative umbrella; and third, many non-traditional sources were used for referrals including pharmacists, churches and business people.

Developing and nurturing support groups is essential because, as noted earlier, their use enhances well-being and is associated with the making of residential plans. Because parents who participate in support groups become advocates and also reach out to other similar families, they are readily recruitable as ancillary outreach persons. Yet, it was evident in our recruitment of respondents, that support groups did not exist in many areas, even where mothers said that they would welcome support from peers. Unless initiatives are made by professionals, support groups may not be formed.

Senior centers and area agency network personnel who are providing services to adults with MR should recruit their parents for MR/DD counselors who can assist them in permanency planning. Fortunately, the proposed 1992 amendments to the Older Americans Act of 1965 call for the provision of services to "older individuals who provide uncompensated care to their adult children with disabilities, or counseling to assist such older individuals with permanency planning for such children" (Congressional Record–House, April 9, 1992, p. 2606). But given the specialized nature of counseling these parents that includes knowledge of alternative living arrangements, referrals should generally be made to MR/DD counselors rather than using aging network personnel as counselors to these families. The provision of personal care services to the parents as they become frail is essential; otherwise the parents become the receivers of care from their offspring, often at the expense of their offspring. Witnessing this reversal exacerbates the feeling among case managers that parents are selfish and trade off their own needs for the needs of the offspring.

Outreach by MR/DD staff is imperative. Because of the resistance to approach counselors regarding making future plans, it is essential that knowledgeable, sensitive MR/DD staff initiate contact with families, particularly to those parents who do not use or under-utilize available services. Among our 235 mothers were 59 who were not currently using day programming services for their off-spring (therapeutic day programs, workshops or competitive employment). In turn, of the 59, 37 had never used day programming services; and because of their purposive avoidance of available services and their self-isolation, must be approached cautiously. The other 22 who had withdrawn their offspring from use of day programs claiming abrasive interactions with staff, reported less family cohesion suggesting generally conflictful relationships. These parents must be approached even more gingerly than those who have never used day programs

COUNSELING

Before focusing on counseling issues *per se* it is essential to understand how the MR/DD system has responded to consumer advocates; that is, advocates have argued that the system should empower the developmentally disabled rather than treat them as clients (Singer & Irvin, 1991). Parents in this paradigm, in turn, are seen as enablers who too easily infantilize their offspring. Yet, elderly parents must be perceived as clients, or potential clients who will become clients, if they are to be helped to overcome their resistance to making permanent residential plans.

Case managers are aware of the emphasis on empowerment and also how the system's focus on quick outcomes hinders the necessary pacing in approaching and then addressing planning for the future. It is, however, essential to go slowly and gingerly. Whereas pacing is always important in counseling, it is especially important to this group who resist planning. It takes time and clinical acumen to develop the trust necessary to overcome resistance.

There is also a need to work with parents whose offspring are in group homes or living independently. To be sure, it is not only those older parents who live with a disabled son or daughter who are distraught over the prospect of their offspring's future. For example, in a focus group conducted by the first author, an older father whose physically disabled daughter lives away from her parents in a setting with similarly disabled women poignantly made the following statement to express his never-ending concern for his daughter's future well being:

> One day, when my wife, my daughter, and I were sitting together and talking, I said to my daughter: 'What if I had a gun and I shot you, then your mother, and then me; Don't you think that would solve all of our concerns about the future?' Well, to my surprise, she looked at me and replied: 'You and mom can shoot yourselves if you wish, but I want to go on living as long as I can.'

As this quote so dramatically illustrates, even those older parents who do have definite residential plans in place for their offspring cannot die peacefully because of their extreme fear that their disabled offspring will not survive without their constant vigilance.

Clinicians must obviously be sensitive to the plight of parents; to the resistance to aging and to acceptance of their deaths from the awareness that permanent residential plans should be made. Their perception of the selfishness of parents who refuse to make these plans may be accurate but obviously must not be communicated. And they must understand that it is not a distortion by parents to perceive care by others after their deaths not to be as good as their care. Yet, sometimes it may be akin to the mother's care when another child who has been especially close to the offspring with MR makes a home in the future. Too often, however, plans made become unmade as the child who has offered to provide a home in the future has a change in life circumstances such as marriages, illness of a spouse or widowhood. Many of our mothers communicated their anxiety regarding how these kinds of potential events would void the contract made between them and their children. One mother who had not discussed the contract with her child, since it was made 28 years ago, apparently had thoughts of the possible changes in her child causing recurrent anxiety.

Diminishing the frustration and anger of clinicians is not at all easy because of countertransference issues. All parents of adults wish their children well but also can feel that they are not doing enough for them. Then, when parents of offspring with MR are selfish, it can evoke feelings in case managers that are better suppressed than felt. In turn, anger toward oneself can readily be deflected toward these parents who indeed can be criticized for not making residential plans for the future; and, also, possibly when having to make abrupt, inadequate plans if the offspring appears on their doorsteps late on a Friday afternoon.

Other children, siblings of the offspring with MR, should be included in the counseling on permanency planning. Most of these parents have other children; only 28 of the 235 did not. Whether other children have agreed or not agreed to make a home, it is important to include them when working with parents. They are an invaluable resource for parents who even if they are not making a future home for their siblings can, and usually do, assume financial arrangements and guardianship.

OTHER INITIATIVES

Must permanent residential placement await the death of parents? Should not, that is, parents consider placing their offspring in the most appropriate settings before their deaths? If so, this is indeed a controversial recommendation because lifelong caring parents have learned how to cope with their disabled offspring, have provided a gratifying normal life at home, and cannot perceive any other place as better. Is this not, in turn, a recommendation to tamper with home and family? Yet Rinck and Calkin's (in press) data on family satisfaction with services indicate satisfaction at the overt level with out-of-home residential placements. Group homes permit normalization of peer relationships and greater autonomy than the interdependence that can develop as aging parents become ill and rely on their offspring for their care. Also, when adult children leave home, intimacy with them does not end. The tradeoff for parents is acceptance of an out-of-home setting perceived as less a home but with possibly diminished fear that their deaths will eventuate in adverse effects on their offspring. Of importance for counseling, Heller and Factor (1991) found that greater use of formal services, including case management, increased the likelihood of a residential placement, a group home, rather than placement with other children.

We would be remiss if another kind of initiative went unrecognized. M. M. Seltzer (1992) has trained families to be case managers for older persons with developmental disabilities. The fragmentation of health and social services for persons aging with disabilities is quite evident (Braddock, 1987). To be sure, professional case management has much to offer but, as observed by M. M. Seltzer (1992), "There are advantages in training family members to participate with professionals in the case management process" (page 65).

Family members who provide direct care and supervision are also in the best position to advocate and monitor services (Fiedler and Antonak, 1991). By training families as case managers, services can be better coordinated with informal care (see especially Silverstone and Burack-Weiss, 1983). M. M. Seltzer and Mayer (1988) have developed the Family Centered Community Care for the Elderly model that appears equally applicable to families caring for members aging with developmental disabilities as to families caring for members who do not have these disabilities.

NOT TO BE FORGOTTEN

Older parents caring for adult aging offspring with developmental disabilities could have been forgotten in the past. They cannot now, however, because advances in medical science and care for chronic illnesses have made these families ubiquitous. Unless we attend to the parents' needs, neither will services benefit them and their offspring nor will the future of their offspring be assured for the times after their deaths. Counselors have an indispensable role in assuring this comfortable future because of the resistance of parents to making permanency plans. Only then, by sensitive and knowledgeable counselors, will those too easily forgotten receive the best we have to offer.

REFERENCES

Braddock, D. (1987). *Federal Policy Toward Mental Retardation and Developmental Disabilities*. Baltimore, MD: Paul H. Brookes.

Brody, E.M. (1985). Parent care as a normative stress. *The Gerontologist, 25,* 19-29.

Carswell, A.T., & Hartig, S.A. (1979). *Older Developmentally Disabled Persons: An Investigation of Needs and Social Services.* Athens: Georgia Retardation Center, Athens Unit, University of Georgia.

Fiedler, C.R., & Antonak, R.F. (1991). Advocacy. In J.L. Matson and J.A. Mulick, Eds., *Handbook of Mental Retardation.* NY: Pergamon Press.

Heller, T., & Factor, A. (1991). Permanency planning for adults with mental retardation living with family caregivers. *American Journal on Mental Retardation, 96,* 163-176.

Horne (1989). Identifying a "hidden" population of older adults with mental handicap: Outreach in the UK. *Australia and New Zealand Journal of Developmental Disabilities, 15,* 207-218.

Janicki, M.P., & Wisniewski, H.M. (1985). *Aging and Developmental Disabilities: Issues and Approaches.* Baltimore, MD: Paul H. Brookes Publishing Co.

Jennings, J. (1987). Elderly parents as caregivers for their adult dependent children. *Social Work, 32,* 430-433.

Kaufman, A.V., DeWeaver, K., & Glicken, M. (1989). The mentally retarded aged: Implications for social work practice. *Journal of Gerontological Social Work, 14,* 93-110.

Lefly, H.P. (1987). Aging parents as caregivers of mentally ill adult children: An emerging social problem. *Hospital and Community Psychiatry, 38,* 1063-1070.

Lieberman, M.A., & Tobin, S.S. (1983). *The Experience of Old Age: Stress, Coping and Survival.* New York: Basic Books.

Lippman, L., & Loberg, D.E. (1985). An overview of developmental disabilities. In M.P. Janicki & H.M. Wisniewski (Eds.), *Aging and Developmental Disabilities: Issue and Approaches.* Baltimore, MD: Paul H. Brookes Publishing Co.

Lubin, R.A., & Kiely, M. (1985). Epidemiology of aging in developmental disabilities. In M.P. Janicki & H.M. Wisniewski (Eds.), *Aging and Developmental Disabilities: Issues and Approaches.* Baltimore, MD: Paul H. Brookes Publishing Co.

Neugarten, B.L., Havighurst, R.J., & Tobin, S.S. (1961). The measurement of life satisfaction, *Journal of Gerontology, 16,* 134-143.

Rinck, C., & Calkins, C.F. (In Press). Family satisfaction with case management and service provision: Rural and urban perspectives for older families of persons with developmental disabilities. In K.A. Roberto (Ed.), *Elderly Caregivers of Developmentally Disabled Adults: Research and Practice.* Beverly Hills, CA: Sage.

Roberto, K.A. (1989). *Caring for aging developmentally disabled adults: Perspectives and needs of older parents.* Final report to the Colorado Developmental Disabilities Planning Council.

Seltzer, M.M. (1992). Training families to be case managers for elders with developmental disabilities. *Generations, 16,* 65-70.

Seltzer, M.M., & Mayer, J.B. (1988). Families as case managers: A team approach for serving the elderly. *Generations, 12,* 26-29.

Seltzer, M.M., & Seltzer, G.B. (1985). The elderly mentally retarded: A group in need of service. *Journal of Gerontological Social Work, 8,* 99-119.

Silverstone, B., & Burack-Weiss, A. (1983). *Social Work Practice with the Frail Elderly and their Families. The Auxiliary Function Model.* Springfield, IL: Thomas.

Singer, G.H.S., & Irvin, L.V. (1991). Supporting families of persons with severe disabilities: Emerging findings, practices and questions. In L.N. Meyer, C.A. Peck & L. Brown (Eds.), *Critical Issues in the Lives of People with Severe Disabilities.* Baltimore: Paul H. Brookes.

Sison, G.F.P., & Cotten, P.D. (1989). The elderly mentally retarded person: Current perspectives and future directions. *The Journal of Applied Gerontology, 8,* 151-167.

Slater, M.A., & Wikler, L. (1986). Normalized family resources for families with a developmentally disabled child. *Social Work, 31,* 385-389.

Smith, G.C., Fullmer, E.M., & Tobin, S.S. (In Press). Living outside the system: An exploration of families who do not use day care. In M.M. Seltzer, M.W. Krauss, & M. Janicki (Eds.), *Life Span Development and Mental Retardation: Implications for Individuals, Their Families and The Human Service System.* Washington, DC: American Association on Mental Retardation.

Smith, G.C., & Tobin, S.S. (1989). Permanency planning among older parents of adults with lifelong disabilities. *Journal of Gerontological Social Work, 14,* 35-59.

Smith, G.C., & Tobin, S.S. (In Press). Case managers' perceptions of practice with older parents of developmentally disabled adults. In K.A. Roberto (Ed.), *Elderly Caregivers of Developmentally Disabled Adults: Research and Practice.* Beverly Hills, CA: Sage.

Smith, G.C., Smith, M.F., & Toseland, R.W. (1991). Problems identified by family caregivers in counseling. *The Gerontologist, 31,* 15-22.

Sutton, E., Sterns, H.L., Schwartz, L., & Roberts, R. (1992). The training of a specialist in developmental disabilities and aging. *Generations, 16,* 71-74.

Tobin, S.S. (1991). *Personhood in Advanced Old Age: Implications for Practice.* New York: Springer.

Tobin, S.S., & Lieberman, M.A. (1976). *Last Home for the Aged: Critical Implications of Institutionalization.* San Francisco, CA: Jossey-Bass.

Wood, J.B., & Skiles, L.L. (1992). Planning for the transfer of care: Who cares for the developmentally disabled adult when the family can no longer do so? *Generations, 16,* 61-62.

Chapter Six

Facilitating Residential Transitions of Older Adults with Developmental Disabilities

Sharon Jacobson, MA
Nancy P. Kropf, PhD

Editor's Introduction

Jacobson and Kropf follow with the next question about the developmentally disabled: What happens when they grow old, and their parents are no longer around to care for them? How can we help them make the transition into new residential facilities? Kahn and Antonucci's social convoy model represents a useful perspective.

Sharon Jacobson is a doctoral student in the Department of Recreation and Leisure Studies and Nancy P. Kropf is Assistant Director of the Gerontology Center and Assistant Professor in School of Social Work at the University of Georgia.

[Haworth co-indexing entry note]: "Facilitating Residential Transitions of Older Adults with Developmental Disabilities." Jacobson, Sharon, and Nancy P. Kropf. Co-published simultaneously in *Clinical Gerontologist* (The Haworth Press, Inc.) Vol. 14, No. 1, 1993, pp. 79-93; and: *The Forgotten Aged: Ethnic, Psychiatric, and Societal Minorities* (ed: T. L. Brink) The Haworth Press, Inc., 1993, pp. 79-93. Multiple copies of this article/chapter may be purchased from The Haworth Document Delivery Center. Call 1-800-3-HAWORTH (1-800-342-9678) between 9:00 - 5:00 (EST) and ask for DOCUMENT DELIVERY CENTER.

INTRODUCTION

The need to address issues relating to older adults with developmental disabilities is becoming increasingly important. With the "graying" of America, the number of older adults with developmental disabilities has increased substantially (Malone, 1990). This population has grown from an estimated population of 350,000 in 1970 (Malone, 1990) to approximately 1,577,340[1] in 1989 (U. S. Census Bureau, 1991). Advances in the provision of health care have been a major factor in the increased life expectancies for all individuals with developmental disabilities (DiGiovanni, 1978; Malone, 1990; Walz, Harper, and Wilson, 1986).

Besides increased life spans, another related issue involves the shift in service delivery paradigms. The deinstitutionalization movement has been a focal issue faced by older people with developmental disabilities, their communities, and family systems. The movement away from restrictive residential living arrangements has triggered a series of structural changes within the social support constellations of these older adults. One disruptive consequence of deinstitutionalization is the expectation that individuals with developmental disabilities will be transferred to a less restrictive environment as their level of competency changes (Krauss and Erickson, 1988; O'Connor, 1983). Frequently, established relationships between older people with developmental disabilities do not factor into decisions about their living arrangements (O'Connor, 1983).

The challenge for professionals who work with this population is to increase the awareness and understanding about the effects of residential transitions upon older adults with developmental disabilities and their social support systems. To better understand these issues, some cogent questions have been raised regarding the effect of residential transitions on the lives of individuals with developmental disabilities (O'Connor, 1983). Does the individual have to start all over each time a residential move occurs? What happens to the person's social support networks including the friends and other supporters left behind? What can agencies do to help ameliorate the stress that stems from this situation for these people? Unfortunately, the answers to these questions frequently are not included in decisions about residential relocations.

This chapter will explore residential transitions for older adults with developmental disabilities. Through a review of the literature and the presentation of a case study, the concept of a social convoy will be introduced, the impact of residential transitions on the social convoy will be presented, and recommendations will be offered how service providers can reduce the negative impact of residential transition on older adults with a developmental disability.

SOCIAL SUPPORT AND RESIDENTIAL TRANSITIONS

The conceptual framework for this study is based on three assumptions. First, the social convoy is a vehicle through which social support is exchanged across the life span in a dynamic and reciprocal manner and whose construction is based on personal constructs and role definitions. Second, older adults with developmental disabilities have a social convoy which has differences and similarities to the general population of older adults. Finally, residential transitions influence the construction of individuals' social convoys. The literature supports the importance of the relationship between the existence and construction of individuals' social convoy and their adaptation to residential transition.

Social Convoy Model

The term social convoy is used to describe a blanket of family and friends who travel through an individual's life course helping them to maneuver through the challenges and celebrate the triumphs (Antonucci and Akiyama, 1987). Social convoys "are thought to be dynamic and lifelong in nature, that is, changing in some ways but remaining stable in others, across time and situations" (Antonucci and Akiyama, 1987, p. 519). Furthermore, through social convoys an individual can give and receive emotional, cognitive, and material support. Social convoys are three tiered in nature, offering a variety of *substantive* supports through an ever changing *spatial* network across *the life span* (Kahn and Antonucci, 1980).

The theoretical framework of the social convoy has been por-

trayed as an image of three concentric circles each of which sur-
round an individual over his or her lifespan (Kahn and Antonucci,
1980). In the model, each circle represents the degree of closeness
shared by the supports (See Figure 1). The individuals who are
members of the inner circle are those people with whom the individual feels extremely close, are independent of the roles that they
play in their lives, and with whom relationships are likely to remain
stable. Examples of these relationships are spouses, close family

FIGURE 1. Hypothetical example of a convoy.

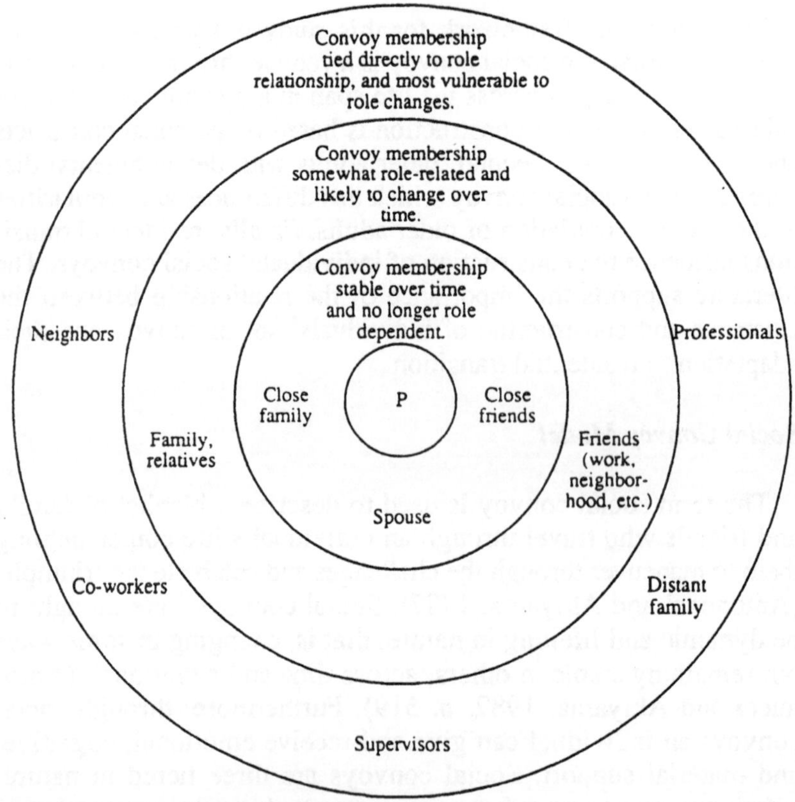

Convoy membership
tied directly to role
relationship, and most vulnerable to
role changes.

Convoy membership
somewhat role-related and
likely to change over
time.

Convoy membership
stable over time
and no longer role
dependent.

Neighbors

Professionals

Close
family

P

Close
friends

Family,
relatives

Friends
(work,
neighbor-
hood, etc.)

Spouse

Co-workers

Distant
family

Supervisors

Permission has been granted to reprint Figure 1 from an article appearing
in *Life Span Development and Behavior*, Volume 3 1980 by the Academic
Press.

and friends. People who are members of the second concentric circle have close relationships with the individual, however, the relationships are based to some extent on a role-prescribed relationship and are susceptible to termination upon loss or change in role. Neighbors, family, in-laws, friends, coworkers, are examples of the types of relationships found in this second circle. The members of the outer circle have relationships with the individual that are totally role dependent. This level might include supervisors, coworkers, neighbors, teachers, and clients.

Construction of an individual's social convoy is dynamic in nature. Changes to the construction of an individual's social convoy may occur in many ways (See Figure 2). Movements in and out of the second and third circles may occur because of transitions in roles, geographic locations, and changes in status of relationships. Changes to the first circle may occur because of death or upon instances of significant betrayal. As people age, the structure of the social convoy begins to shrink due to increased mortality, increased role loss, and geographic relocation.

Reciprocity is an important characteristic of the social convoy. While it is important for individuals to receive support, people also need to be valued and helpful to others. The relationships that exist at any given point in time provide a vehicle through which an individual may both receive and offer social support.

People have individual ways of assessing the degree of closeness in their social convoy (Jacobson, 1987; Kahn and Antonucci, 1980). Therefore, individuals' social convoy may vary from no members in a given circle to many members in another level circle. For example, one individual may describe her social convoy as consisting of many role dependent relationships and only one person with whom she has a significantly close relationship. This example would describe an older person who is involved with several service providers (clergy, physicians, social worker) but has only one close family or friendship relationship. A second individual may describe his convoy as having few role dependent relationships and several significantly close relationships. This situation would describe an older man who is part of a close family and neighborhood and does not use formal services. Social convoys differ in the number of and degree of closeness to persons with whom supportive relationships

FIGURE 2. Changing convoy composition over the life course: one woman's convoy at two different points in her life cycle.

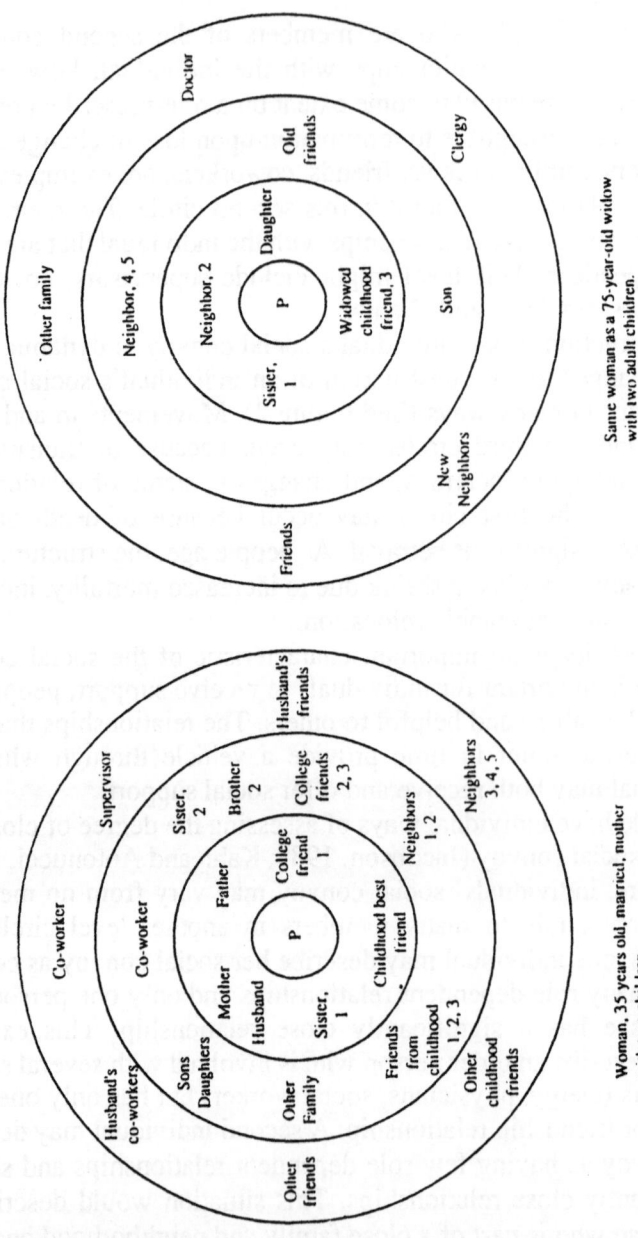

Woman, 35 years old, married, mother with two children.

Same woman as a 75-year-old widow with two adult children.

Permission has been granted to reprint Figure 2 from an article appearing in *Life Span Development and Behavior*, Volume 3 1980 by the Academic Press.

are maintained. Both the existence and size of a social convoy are predictors of well-being and of the ability to cope successfully with stress (Kahn and Antonucci, 1980).

Social Support of Older Adults
with Developmental Disabilities

The benefit of social support and the importance of the social convoy in providing support for older adults is well documented. Members of an individual's social convoy provide many physical and mental health benefits such as reducing the impact of age re-lated functional changes, maintaining lifestyles, deterring negative aspects of grief, and increasing social interaction (Adams, 1985; Chappell, 1983; Jacobson, 1987). While the benefits of a social convoy are of equal benefit to older adults with developmental disabilities, the opportunity to develop supportive relationships is different (Boyd and Tedrick, 1992). People with disabilities face limited social and economic opportunities in which they develop social support systems.

The social support that is exchanged through the social convoy is important to all older adults both with and without developmental disabilities. Krauss and Erickson (1988) in their study of the social convoys of older adults with developmental disabilities identified " . . . the critical role of peer relationships in the informal support networks of aging persons with mental retardation" (p. 200). So-cial convoys of older adults with developmental disabilities differ by residential living arrangement. People residing in non-family settings had social convoys that consisted mainly of friends and professionals. These differed from those living in family settings whose convoys consisted primarily of family (Boyd and Tedrick, 1992; Krauss and Erickson, 1988; Willer and Intagliata, 1981). The convoys of older people with developmental disabilities are heavily influenced by their type of living arrangement, as supports are often based on proximity.

Losses and disruptions to a social convoy may result in a variety of negative changes to one's physical, emotional, and social behav-iors. Disruption of older adults' social convoy may result in an increase in mortality (Danermark and Ekstrom, 1990), pessimism (Bourestom and Tars, 1974), decreased social behavior (Bourestom and Tars, 1974), mental health capacities, self care, and health problems (Danermark and Ekstrom, 1990; Miller and Lieberman, 1965). While these losses and disruptions have received little attention as they affect older adults with developmental disabilities, Krauss and Erickson (1988) suggest that loss or disruption of a social convoy may generate a depressive state for an older person with a developmental disability. Losses in support for this population may be magnified since many people with developmental disabilities have limited opportunities to replenish support systems.

Residential Transition of Older Adults with Developmental Disabilities

One way that social convoys are disrupted is through relocations and moves. As a group, people with developmental disabilities are susceptible to abrupt residential moves. The frequency with which residential transitions occur varies with residential placement. Krauss and Erickson (1988) reported that individuals over age 40 who lived in community residential placement had been relocated 4.1 times, individuals who were living in institutional settings had been relocated an average of 2.9 times, and those who resided at home had no prior placements. Clearly, older people with developmental disabilities who reside outside the family home are most likely to experience residential changes.

Residential transition does not just impact the individual, it affects the family, friends, and the agencies. Friends, family, and other caregivers constitute the social convoy that provides support to older adults (Adams, 1985; Boyd and Tedrick, 1992; Krauss and Erickson, 1988; O'Connor, 1983). What happens to them then when the individual moves? Part of the social convoy model involves both receiving and providing support. Rarely, are the consequences to those "left behind" considered in residential relocation decisions.

For older adults, with and without developmental disabilities, the effect of relocation can be especially traumatic. The relocation of an older adult to a new residential setting disrupts the perceptions and feelings about one's environment and established relationships (Danermark and Ekstrom, 1990; O'Connor, 1983; Rubenstein, 1989). These losses include the unique roles held by the older person in that situation and a perception of control and mastery in that environment (Berciovici 1981; Heller 1982; Krauss and Erickson 1988). For example, an older woman with mental retardation may be viewed as the "grandmother" figure to younger adults in one residential setting. If she moves to a placement with all older people, she would lose her unique role, as in the following case study.

Case Study: Janet Houseman

The following case study provides an example of a residential relocation for an older woman with mental retardation, Janet Houseman. The information is used to exemplify the consequences of relocation both for Janet and her supports.

Janet Houseman is a 61-year old woman with mental retardation. She has resided in an institution in a small southern town since she was 12. Since her admittance, she has had virtually no contact with her family.

Janet has many functional abilities. She can dress, feed, use the bathroom independently, and has good verbal skills. On Janet's wing, she lives with younger adults who have lower degrees of functional abilities. Janet has made friends with two of the other women (both in their 30s) and she is involved in assisting them with their needs. They have struck a good friendship and Janet values spending time with them. The three women have lived together on the same wing for about twelve years.

Due to Janet's tenure at the institution, she also has made some long-standing relationships with staff. While many staff work only a short time, one social worker has known Janet for many years. Although the social worker has been promoted and works elsewhere, she comes over to see Janet about twice a month for lunch or coffee.

Janet has been in fairly good health all her life yet she is now beginning to display some age-related changes. She is having a difficult time walking due to some arthritis in her joints. This condition presents problems getting around in the institution and on one occasion she fell in the hallway. The problem is exacerbated by decreased eyesight and some hearing loss.

The treatment team is concerned about Janet's conditions and her ability to continue to function in the institution. Her team felt that they were neither equipped nor staffed to handle Janet's emerging chronic care needs. They investigated a residential relocation to a facility that specializes in the geriatric population. An adult foster care home, located about 30 miles away, was willing to accept Janet. This home currently houses four older women who have some type of chronic impairment. The team thought this move would be a good one, since Janet could be with other older women.

Janet was moved into the foster care home a short time later. Although Janet was informed about the move, she was only given three days notice when the final date was scheduled. The staff packed up her belongings, and two aides drove her to the new residence. The new staff escorted her to her room and unpacked her belongings.

Soon after the move, she began exhibiting some adjustment problems. The other women were older and they would talk about their grandchildren which would exclude Janet. Although she could call her two friends on the telephone, neither of them had good verbal skills so there was limited conversation. Although she had a room of her own, she didn't want to stay in there at night since all of her life she had shared a room with others. She spent most of her day in the bathroom, where she would cry for hours.

RECOMMENDATIONS FOR PRACTICE

This case exemplifies problems with residential relocations of older adults with developmental disabilities. Often decisions about relocations are made quickly, without time to transition from one place to another. In the case of Janet, she was relocated to a new environment that was less structured than the institution. This situation was unfamiliar and frightening and there was no time to help her build skills to adjust to her new surroundings. Additionally, there was limited time for her to say goodbye to the people who were important to her in the institution.

The trauma of residential relocation of older people with mental retardation can be decreased if multi-level interventions are planned around the move. First, preparations need to be planned to help the person who will be relocating. The individual should be included in the planning and decision making process whenever possible. A second consideration is the effect of the residential change on the members of the social convoy who are "left behind." In Janet's case, she has left some significant relationships with people in the institution. She has shared close ties with the two younger women on her floor, as well as the social worker who has become a friend figure to her. The third level of intervention in residential transition is preparing the new environment. These plans include both physical and social arrangements. The development and implementation of transitional plans are critical in facilitating the impact of residential transition for the older adult with a developmental disability. These plans are especially important for individuals with mental retardation because of their limited ability for abstract thinking.

Preparing the Individual

As illustrated in the case study of Janet, numerous opportunities existed to facilitate her residential transition. One consideration is to understand the skills that Janet required to function in the new environment and ways to help her build those before the residential change. One issue for Janet, who had spent 46 years sharing a room with someone, was the adjustment to a private room. Transitional living plans would have permitted Janet to master the skills of being by herself at night. One method of helping Janet adapt would have been to have her attempt a single room at the institution, a familiar environment.

Pre-placement visits to the foster care home also would have reduced her anxiety and made the move less drastic. Janet could have been allowed to pack and unpack her belongings or at least be a part of the process (Harkulich and Brugler, 1991). Arrangements to continue her monthly lunch with her former social worker would have allowed Janet to stay connected to an important member of her social convoy.

Preparing the Members of Her Social Convoy

A departure also has an impact on the social convoy members "left behind." Relationships with staff at the former facility are normally severed. Friends left behind lose a friend and the support that the person provided to them. The move also leaves gaps in their social convoys. Steps could be taken to prepare for the individuals who will remain at the residential setting.

In Janet's case, relationships with former staff and residents could have continued through visits at the new residence. The former social worker could have continued to schedule planned lunches at the new facility. Her two young friends could have been involved in the moving process of both packing and unpacking of Janet's possessions. These steps allow her friends to be a part of the excitement of moving to a new environment. Unfortunately, low priority is often placed on ways to enable friends to remain connected by visiting other residences.

For people with mental retardation, creativity is needed in helping friends remain in contact. Due to the limited verbal skills of the young women at the institution, telephone conversations did not promote their continued contact with Janet. This situation could be resolved using video or photographic messages.

Staff also should support those left behind to ensure that they do not experience feelings of guilt or abandonment over the move (Harkulich and Brugler, 1991). The use of a "celebration" event such as a going away party to mark the change of location also would allow for more direct involvement of those who have the closest relationships to the person. In Janet's case, her two younger friends and the social worker may have a planned relocation party to help celebrate her stay at the institution. Unfortunately, the life stages of people with mental retardation often "bleed" into each other without the benefit of rituals that mark different phases such as graduations, wedding ceremonies, and retirement parties. These events are beneficial for individuals who are relocating and the social convoy members who feel involved in ushering in a new life phase.

Preparing the New Environment

The individuals at the new residence need to be prepared for the change in their environment. Many steps can be taken to prepare the social environment for a new person. Residential meetings can be held to inform the residents about the newcomer, and to share important information about the person between service providers. In Janet's situation, the older women could have been informed about Janet's history and experiences that are different from those of the other residents. Staff from both facilities can exchange information about the individual to insure there is consistency and continuity in care delivery (Harkulich and Brugler, 1991) such as knowing Janet's favorite foods, her likes and dislikes, and her routines.

Besides the social environment, physical modifications can help with the transition phase. For people with mental retardation, this process may need to include identifying unfamiliar objects and territories of the residents. For example, a picture of each woman could be posted on her bedroom door to initially identify each of the residents' rooms for Janet. For people familiar to institutional environments, there may be a lack of competence in areas mastered by non-retarded individuals. People with mental retardation often have not gained mastery over skills common in the community such as pedestrian skills, or interacting with animals such as pet dogs and cats. The environment needs to be evaluated to address specific age-related needs and those related to the developmental disability of new residents.

CONCLUSION

Through the inclusion of steps such as those discussed above, the older adult with a developmental disability can receive support and assistance with their residential changes. Since many people with mental retardation experience relocations, often enacted abruptly, suggestions have been proposed to ameliorate the stress. These steps involve preparation for the older individuals, their supports, and the new environment.

Individuals who will be relocated need to be involved in their move as much as possible. This process makes the residential shift less dramatic and promotes a sense of empowerment for the older adult. Members of the older adult's social convoy also need to be prepared for relocation changes. These individuals can participate in the relocation process and be helped to supplement their own support systems that also will be affected by the move. Additionally, the new environment needs to be assessed to address the physical and social needs of an older person with mental retardation.

ENDNOTE

1. This figure was derived using 3% of the total population of age 55 and over to remain consistent with cited population estimates from 1970.

REFERENCES

Adams, R. G. (1985). Emotional closeness and physical distance between friends: Implications for elderly women living in age-segregated and age-integrated settings. *International Journal of Aging and Human Development*, 22(1), 55-76.

Antonucci, T. C. and Akiyama, H. (1987). Social networks in adult life and a preliminary examination of the convoy model. *Journal of Gerontology*, 42(5), 519-527.

Berciovici, S. M. (1981). Qualitative methods in cultural perspectives in the study of deinstitutionalization. In Bruininks, R. H., Meyers, C. E., Sigford, B. B., and Lakin, K. C. (Eds.). *Deinstitutionalization and community adjustment of mentally retarded people.* (Monograph No 4). Washington, DC: American Academy on Mental Deficiency.

Bourestom, N. C. and Tars, S. (1974). Alterations in life patterns following nursing home relocation. *The Gerontologist*, 14, 506-510.

Boyd, R. and Tedrick, T. (1992). Aging adults with mental retardation and leisure. *Parks and Recreation*, 27(10), 20-27, 86.

Chappell, N. L. (1983). Informal support networks among the elderly. *Research on Aging*, 5(1), 77-99.

Danermark, B. and Ekstrom, M. (1990). Relocation and health effects on the elderly: A commented research review. *Journal of Sociology and Social Welfare*, 17(1), 25-49.

DiGiovanni, L. (1978). The elderly retarded: A little known group. *The Gerontologist*, 18(3), 262-266.

Harkulich, J. T. and Brugler, C. (1991). Relocation and the resident. *Activities, Adaptation, and Aging*, 16, 51-60.

Heller, T. (1982). Social disruption and residential relocation of mentally retarded children. *American Journal of Mental Retardation*, 87(1), 48-55.

Jacobson, D. (1987). The cultural context of social support and support networks. *Medical Anthropology Quarterly*, 1(1), 42-67.

Kahn, R. L. and Antonucci, T. C. (1980). Convoys over the life course: Attachment, roles and support. In Baltes, P. B. and Brim, O. G. (Eds.), *Life Span Development and Behavior*, Volume 3. New York: Academic Press.

Krauss, M. W. and Erickson, M. (1988). Informal support networks among aging persons with mental retardation: A pilot study. *Mental Retardation*, 26(4), 197-201.

Malone, M. (1990). Aging persons with mental retardation: Identification of the needs of a special population. *Gerontology Review*, 3(1), 1-14.

Miller, D. and Liebermann, M. A. (1965). The relationship of affect state and adaptive capacity to reactions to stress. *Journal of Gerontology*, 20, 492-497.

O'Connor, G. (1983). Presidential address 1983: Social support of mentally retarded persons. *Mental Retardation, 21*(5), 187-196.

Rubenstein, R. L. (1989). The home environments of older people: A description of the psychosocial processes linking person to place. *Journal of Gerontology, 44*(2), S45-53.

U. S. Bureau of Census. (1991). *Statistical abstracts of the United States: 1991* (111th edition). Washington, DC: U. S. Government Printing Office.

Walz, T., Harper, D., and Wilson, J. (1986). The aging developmentally disabled person: A review. *The Gerontologist, 26*(6), 622-629.

Willer, B. and Intagliata, J. (1981). Socio-environmental factors as predictors of adjustment of deinstitutionalized mentally retarded adults. 252-259.

Chapter Seven

Mental Health Outreach to Rural Elderly: Service Delivery to a Forgotten Risk Group

Diane G. Snustad, MD
Anita A. Thompson-Heisterman, RN, MS, CS
Jane B. Neese, RN, MS, CS
Ivo L. Abraham, RN, PhD, FAAN

Editor's Introduction

Snustad et al. explore the special challenges confronting a multi-disciplinary team attempting mental health outreach for

---

Diane G. Snustad is Assistant Professor, Department of Medicine and Department of Behavioral Medicine and Psychiatry; and Assistant Director of Clinical Programs, Center on Aging and Health, University of Virginia. Anita A. Thompson-Heisterman is Clinical Assistant Professor, Jefferson Area Rural Elder Health Consortium, Center on Aging and Health, University of Virginia. Jane B. Neese is a W. K. Kellogg Foundation Fellow, Center on Aging and Health, NRSA Fellow, National Institutes of Health, and a doctoral candidate, University of Virginia. Ivo L. Abraham is Associate Professor of Nursing, Associate Professor of Behavioral Medicine and Psychiatry, Director, Center on Aging and Health, and Co-Director, Southeastern Rural Mental Health Research Center, University of Virginia. He is also Professor of Nursing, Health Policy and Health Administration at the Catholic University of Leuven, Leuven, Belgium.

[Haworth co-indexing entry note]: "Mental Health Outreach to Rural Elderly: Service Delivery to a Forgotten Risk Group." Snustad, Diane G. et al. Co-published simultaneously in *Clinical Gerontologist* (The Haworth Press, Inc.) Vol. 14, No. 1, 1993, pp. 95-111; and: *The Forgotten Aged: Ethnic, Psychiatric, and Societal Minorities* (ed: T. L. Brink) The Haworth Press, Inc., 1993, pp. 95-111. Multiple copies of this article/chapter may be purchased from The Haworth Document Delivery Center. Call 1-800-3-HAWORTH (1-800-342-9678) between 9:00 - 5:00 (EST) and ask for DOCUMENT DELIVERY CENTER.

rural elders. The authors' approach should serve as a model, not only for clinical gerontologists working with rural elders, but also with other segments of the forgotten aged.

Over a decade ago, the Panel on Rural Health of the President's Commission of Mental Health (1978) stated, "Rural communities tend to be characterized by higher than average rates of psychiatric disorders, particularly depression, by severe intergenerational conflicts, by restricted opportunities for developing adequate coping mechanisms for facing stress and for problem solving, by an exodus of individuals who might serve as effective role models for coping, by an acceptance of conditions as being beyond individual control, and by acceptance of fatalistic attitudes and minimal subscription to the idea that change is possible" (Pg. 1164; quoted in Buckwalter et al., 1988). Although this statement referred to all age groups, it is most pertinent to the rural elderly population, in which prevalence rates of manifested psychiatric problems have been reported between 23% (Scheidt & Windely, 1982) and 25% (Rosen, Coppage, Troglin, & Rosen, 1981). Considering that more than eight million people over the age of 65 (or 25% of the older population) live in rural America, at least two million rural elderly may be in need of mental health services.

These figures only reflect psychiatric illnesses and do not consider other mental health issues in the elderly: psychiatric/behavioral manifestations of physical illnesses, physical manifestations of psychiatric illnesses, and psychological adaptation to physical illnesses. These additional mental health problems, for which epidemiological data are absent, only add to the complexity of geriatric mental health issues among rural elderly.

Despite the need for rural geriatric mental health services, the NIMH biannual mental health facility surveys document a paucity of local mental health services in rural areas and few psychiatric beds in general community hospitals (Wagenfeld, 1990). Not only are rural areas less likely to have geriatric services, but when the services are offered, they are generally too narrow in scope to meet the needs of rural elders and their families (Fleming et al., 1988). Programs such as Alzheimer's disease support groups and education programs for caregivers on age-specific issues are almost nonexistent in rural communities. The relative absence of formal geriatric mental health services for rural elderly results in higher utilization of local emergency services regardless of whether these are capable of responding to mental health problems (U. S. Congress, Office of Technology Assessment, 1990). Compounding the lack of programs, but also associated with it, is the shortage of trained health professionals in geriatric mental health (Coward & Lee, 1985). Other barriers to delivering mental health services relate to general lack of knowledge among rural families about mental health and available services, geographic and social isolation, lack of transportation, large catchment areas (encompassing up to 60,000 square miles), concerns about confidentiality, a dearth of suitable service models, and ageism, or relative negative attitudes toward the elderly on the part of health care professionals (Waxman, 1986).

Three additional risk factors add to the complexity of rural geriatric mental health, prevalence rates of problems, and service access and utilization patterns: poverty, minority status, and female gender as well as the interaction of all three. One third of all rural elderly have incomes below the poverty line (U. S. Congress, Office of Technology Assessment, 1990). Poverty is twice as high among rural elderly blacks compared to their white counterparts, with one out of two rural black elders living in poverty (Harper, 1990). Ninety-five percent of minority rural elderly live in the South. In particular, rural elderly women are at risk. Sixty-eight percent of all black elderly women in rural areas live in poverty, as well as 40% of white elderly women (Harper & Alexander, 1990; Abraham et al., in press). Approximately 40% of poor rural elderly do not qualify for Medicaid; therefore, many must supplement their Medicare with private insurance or pay cash, making affordability an obstacle (U.S. Congress, Office of Technology Assessment, 1990).

Mental health care is inaccessible to many rural elderly for not only are there fewer providers, but the closure of many rural physician practices and hospitals has forced rural citizens to seek health care in distant urban areas (U. S. Office of Technology Assessment, 1990). The lack of transportation services particularly puts the rural elderly at a disadvantage, as they often do not have or cannot drive their own car (Palmore, 1983/84). Mental health outreach services are limited to a few demonstration initiatives struggling for permanency and sustainability (Abraham et al., in press; Buckwalter et al., 1991). The personnel needed to maintain functionally and cognitively impaired elders in their home are not available in rural areas (Wagenfeld, 1990).

Due to the lack of accessible medical care, the expense of medical care that is available, and attitudes toward care, the rural elderly often wait longer to seek care, present with more health problems and use home remedies as a first response to illness (Palmore, 1983/84). There is often a delayed identification of urgent and/or complex mental health problems. Because of this, the rural elderly are often admitted to hospitals when they are sicker, have longer lengths of stay in acute care hospitals than urban elderly (Deprez, Pennell, & Libby, 1987) and are discharged to long term care facilities rather than back home due to lack of resources in the community to help the rural elder return home. Rural elders are more at risk of premature institutionalization and those in institutions are found to be younger and functionally less impaired than institutionalized non-rural elderly (Greene, 1984).

Outreach services offer an approach to increasing the equity and accessibility of mental health services to this at-risk vulnerable population (Abraham et al., in press; Buckwalter et al. 1991). One such model is the Jefferson Area Rural Elder Health Outreach Program ("REOP") in Charlottesville, Virginia, a community partnership of the University of Virginia, the Region Ten Community Services Board (the public mental health agency), and the Jefferson Area Board for Aging (the area agency on aging). The overall goal is to meet the health care needs of psychosocially at-risk elder residents of rural areas who do not have adequate access to health services and are at risk for institutionalization in nursing homes or psychiatric institutions, hospitalization in acute care facilities, or inappropriate use of emergency services. Through outreach assessment, case management, caregiver support and community educators, the program aims to link formal community-based services, informal community resources, volunteer efforts and academic resources in order to strengthen the self-reliance of rural communities to care for their elderly citizens (Abraham & Neese, in press; Neese, Abraham, Currie, Smullen, & Thompson-Heisterman, 1992). In addition, the Program serves as a training laboratory for clinicians from several disciplines, offering an environment for learning how to collaborate to meet the needs of this population. Services are provided by a multidisciplinary team of nurses, physicians, and social workers, for which psychogeriatric nurses operate as the focal care provider.

The services that are provided, and the principles that guide these services, are discussed individually below, and illustrated by case studies. Although the program is designed to be appropriate for the epidemiology, demography, topography, social and cultural environment, and economic and resource infrastructure of the rural Southeast, these services and principles can be readily extended to other geographic areas.

MULTIDISCIPLINARY ASSESSMENT AND INTERVENTION

Psychological, physical and social problems of the elderly are closely intertwined and are best evaluated and treated by a multidisciplinary team. In the elderly, psychiatric illness often presents with physical symptoms and vice versa. Presentation of illness and treatment needs are both greatly affected by the client's environment. The elder outreach team consists of a geriatric psychiatrist, geriatrician, nurse clinicians, and social workers. Most outreach is done by nurses with occasional support from a physician when appropriate and needed. Cases are presented and discussed in a formal meeting and plans of treatment are formulated. In this way the expertise of all the members of the team is available to patient and family, but in a cost-effective way because not all the team members need to actually travel the long distances to see the patient.

Case Study–Mr. B.

Mr. B. is an 81-year old white widower who was referred to REOP for evaluation of depression. The nurse clinician's evaluation showed him to be severely depressed with decreased appetite, weight loss, sleep disturbance, anhedonia and dysphoria. He had considered shooting himself, and since his son with whom he lived hunted, the home contained several firearms. During this initial visit, the clinical nurse specialist requested that the son remove all the firearms from the home and made a suicide contract with the patient.

Mr. B.'s case was presented in the multidisciplinary meeting. The consensus was that Mr. B. was suffering from a major depressive disorder. The geriatric psychiatrist later made a home visit with the clinical nurse specialist and then spoke to Mr. B.'s local physician and recommended treatment with sertraline. The geriatrician spoke with the family physician regarding the patient's use of three different benzodiazepines, of which his local physician was unaware. The social worker provided information on Medicaid eligibility and addressed Mr. B.'s financial concerns, which were contributing to his depression. After antidepressive treatment, adjustment of his medication, and psychosocial interventions, Mr. B.'s suicidal ideation disappeared and his mood significantly improved, as evidenced by his Hamilton Depression Scale score dropping from 32 to 6.

INTEGRATING COMMUNITY SERVICES

Community services can be strengthened and expanded by cooperation and coordination among agencies. Like their urban counterparts, rural elders often require a wide range of coordinated services to remain functionally independent. Often many of the services that a client needs are available but either he/she is unaware of them or does not know how to access them. Using the case manager approach, the nurse clinician can coordinate the services of various agencies while also providing the necessary mental health services that are lacking in the current system. This can prevent duplication of services in various agencies, and the communication that is fostered allows greater efficiency. Linkages have been made to the area agency on aging for home delivered meals, home safety assessments and equipment, and socialization through senior nutrition sites and friendly visitors. Referrals to social service agencies have provided evaluation for entitlement, personal care aid assistance and fuel assistance. Referrals have also been made to the area hospice, public health department, home health agencies, local community mental health clinics and to family support groups such as those organized by the Alzheimer's Association. The nurse clinician's relationship with community providers and agencies is a key component of the Rural Elder Outreach Program and assures integration and coordination as well as reducing fragmentation and dispersion of services.

Case Study–Ms. W.

Ms. W. was an 86-year old widowed African-American widow who lived with her 64-year old daughter, E.W. Ms. W. was severely demented from a stroke and had been for several years prior to our intervention. Her daughter, E.W., had been providing all of the care for her mother. Even though caregiving was very important to the daughter's self-concept, she became depressed and was subsequently admitted to a psychiatric in-patient ward for major depression with psychotic features. During this time, the mother was admitted to the hospital as well since there were no other available caregivers. Referral was made to REOP for caregiver support post hospitalization.

After evaluation by the nurse, referrals were made to various community services. The Department of Social Services provided a care aide three days a week to assist E. W. in caring for her mother. The REOP nurse facilitated E. W.'s follow-up at the local mental health center by arranging a referral and transportation. A referral was made for the mother, Ms. W., to the geriatric medicine clinic, since she did not have a primary physician. The daughter was unable to obtain groceries on a regular basis due to lack of available public transportation and the fear of leaving her mother unattended. The REOP nurse coordinated home delivered meals including liquid supplement, as the mother's dentition prevented her from eating solid food. On a few occasions, the REOP nurse picked up and delivered the meals when the area agency on aging did not have a driver for that area of the county. During the summer, the nurse contacted social services to obtain a fan for the family since the home had no air conditioning. The REOP nurse also was involved in educating the daughter on how to care for her demented mother and provided written information to review. The consulting psychiatrist made a home visit to evaluate the mother for psychotropic medication to help manage the hallucinations that contributed to agitated behavior.

ASSURING ACCESS

Rural elderly often encounter psychological, financial and physical barriers to health care. Distrust of traditional medical care, a high rate of illiteracy and poverty, and geographical isolation make access to health care difficult for non-urban elders. Through education, gentle persuasion, interpretation of the health care system, use of available assistance programs and at times direct facilitation, the Rural Elder Outreach Program is frequently successful in helping the elderly overcome these barriers. As the following case study suggests, volunteers can assume an important role in assuring access.

Case Study—Ms. R.

Ms. R. is a 73-year old African-American who lives with her husband in a mobile home on the side of a mountain. She was referred by the area agency on aging for substance abuse counseling, chronic health problems and psychosocial support. She had several health problems, including intermittent severe intestinal pain with substantial weight loss in the previous six months, and poor dentition. She had a pattern of making emergency room visits to the tertiary care center twenty miles from her house. Because of cost and distance, she had not seen a primary physician in several years and did not follow through on appointments she was given in the emergency room.

In addition to providing substance abuse counseling, the clinical nurse specialist was able to convince Ms. R. to see a physician for her abdominal pain. The work-up revealed a polyp in her large intestine, which was successfully removed. The REOP nurse and a program volunteer were able to arrange transportation to appointments, accompany Ms. R. to the appointments, interpret results of the evaluation, and function as her advocate in the maze of the health care system. In addition to coordinating Ms. R.'s medical care, the nurse also assisted her by delivering and explaining diagnostic test preparations, drawing blood for laboratory tests, and doing health and medication teaching. As Ms. R. was functionally illiterate, the nurse interpreted her medical bills. Ms. R. now receives primary medical care from a physician, rather than inappropriately using the emergency room.

COUNSELING

Psychological counseling is a much needed service that is often either not available or not acceptable to the rural elder client. Many rural communities lack formal psychiatric care. When it is available, it is often many miles from a client's home. In addition, psychiatric care is associated with a great stigma in many groups of people, particularly rural dwellers and the elderly. By providing services in the privacy of a client's home, the program fosters acceptance of needed psychological support. Furthermore, the program promotes confidentiality by driving in unmarked cars, and being identified primarily with the local agency on aging, rather than a mental health agency. With these precautions, REOP has been successful in delivering counseling services to clients who either could not or would not avail themselves of these services in the past.

Case Study–Ms. W.

Ms. W. is a 77-year old white married woman who is referred to REOP following hospitalization for a hip fracture. While hospitalized, difficulty swallowing, anorexia, and weight loss with no apparent physical cause were observed. Of note was that these were some of the same symptoms experienced by her son who recently died of intestinal cancer. Prior to his death, Mrs. W. had provided total care for her son, with whom she had always had a close but ambivalent relationship. She never expressed nor resolved her grief regarding his death, although she was able to recognize that the symptoms she had could be related to an expression of this grief.

Brief psychotherapy was provided to Mrs. W. in her home by the clinical nurse specialist with the focus on resolution of the underlying conflicts of the complicated grief reaction. During the twelve week therapy, all of her symptoms abated and she gained back nearly all of the eighteen pounds she had lost during the year after her son died.

CAREGIVER SUPPORT

Caregiving stress is common and support is often lacking in rural communities. Adult day care and caregiver support groups that help relieve caregiver stress in urban areas are rarely available in rural areas. In addition, caregiving stress is greater when patient care services are sparse. Stress related illnesses are frequent among caregivers and the risk exists for breakage of the caregiving bond and subsequent institutionalization. REOP is able to provide support for caregivers through counseling and coordination of available services.

Case Study–Mr. R.

Mr. R. is a 74-year old white married man suffering from dementia. Although he has been able to perform some of his activities of daily living he requires a great deal of care. He has a history of alcohol abuse and at times still abuses over-the-counter medications. He has been physically and verbally abusive of his wife, a 66-year old woman with hypertension which she blames partially on the stress of caregiving.

The nurse clinician provides both support and education for Mrs. R. in her care for the husband. The outreach visits provide a regular opportunity for reducing stress in which Mrs. R. can ventilate feelings and problem solve situations. The nurse helps medically to monitor both Mr. and Mrs. R. and provides information to their primary physician and social workers.

FAMILY COUNSELING

Because the family is so important in the care of a disabled elder, care of the elderly often becomes care of the family. This is especially true in rural areas where the need for linkages to informal care providers is high. Family counseling is another service that is often not available or not acceptable to the rural elderly. Despite this, it is a frequently needed service, especially as the strains of growing older with increasing disabilities often put additional stress on the family relationships. REOP overcomes past financial, psychological and logistic barriers to such counseling by providing free counseling services in the home with a nurse with whom the family has already established a relationship.

Case Study–Mr. G.

Mr. G. is a 77-year old married African-American with a ten year history of Parkinson's disease. He was referred to REOP following a hospitalization for depression and medication-related delirium. Mr. G. and his wife have had long-standing marital discord exacerbated by Mr. G.'s increasing dependence on her secondary to his Parkinson's disease. He has a history of questioning her marital fidelity even though Mrs. G. insists that there has been no cause for this. At times Mr. G. has become frankly delusional, accusing her of adultery and even of having become pregnant by another man.

Though traditional marital therapy is not possible due to Mr. G.'s mental status, the nurse clinician regularly meets with the couple in order to allow them to openly discuss their concerns regarding one another in a forum that allows possible resolution of specific issues. Mrs. G. has been able to discuss her embarrassment about her husband's sharing his accusations with others outside the family. He has been able to share his anger about her using his limited money for household expenses, despite her larger income. This counseling intervention has provided an outlet for the couple, which helps to diffuse the anger that builds up between them. It also enables Mrs. G. to continue the care that Mr. G. requires.

PSYCHIATRIC DIAGNOSIS AND TREATMENT

Evaluation and treatment of psychiatric problems often requires expertise not generally available in rural communities. A typical presentation of diseases, multiple medical problems, and psychosocial factors can all make psychiatric diagnosis a perplexing problem in the elderly. Often the medical services that are available in the rural community have neither the time nor the expertise to fully evaluate complex presentations. REOP provides the time and expertise needed to sort out complex presentations.

Case Study–Ms. C.

Ms. C. is an 80-year old white woman who was referred by her primary physician to REOP for an evaluation of dementia versus depression. Her medical problems included chronic lung disease, arthritis, macular degeneration, hypertension and bilateral mastectomies for breast cancer five years previously. She had become very confused after returning home from a visit to her son in Louisiana. During this trip she had visited the grave of her daughter who had died six years previously. She became very tearful when discussing her daughter's death. Additionally, her chronic shortness of breath had worsened to the point where she was unable to perform simple tasks without becoming dyspneic. She reported anxiety, poor appetite with a fifteen pound weight loss, insomnia which she attributed to her breathing difficulties, but no suicidal ideation. It was discovered that she had theophylline toxicity, which caused confusion and disorientation. Once her theophylline level returned to normal, she showed no evidence of cognitive problems. Work-up for reversible causes of dementia was normal. Computed tomographic scan of the head revealed diffuse cerebral atrophy and periventricular white matter disease. This was interpreted by her family to mean that she had Alzheimer's disease, which caused them considerable distress. The REOP nurse was able to educate them and reassure them that this was not necessarily so. It was also found that she was hypoxic and she was begun on oxygen. The final diagnosis was depression related to unresolved losses and to current attempts to adjust to chronic disability, complicated by delirium related to her theophylline toxicity and hypoxia. She became more functional and the nurse continues to work with her to resolve her grief regarding her losses.

CRISIS INTERVENTION

Rural mental health agencies often lack the staff, resources and education to appropriately handle psychiatric emergencies. Because of lack of funding and difficulty in attracting well trained personnel to rural areas, management of psychiatric emergencies is very difficult. In the rural area served by REOP, there are few services available for emergent crisis intervention in the home. It is typical to have case managers with no formal mental health training and little experience. There is a great need for properly trained personnel, a gap which REOP helps to fill.

Case Study–Ms. R.

Ms. R. is a 67-year old African-American woman with the diagnosis of schizo-affective disorder. She is followed by the community mental health center where she receives monthly injections of fluphenazine decanoate. She began to decompensate because she had not received her medication for two months and there was no one who could go to her home and give it to her. The case manager at the community mental health center requested that the REOP clinical nurse specialist evaluate the client for possible hospitalization. Upon arrival at Ms. R.'s home it was discovered that she had placed many of her belongings in her yard, saying that she planned to bring these things with her to the hospital. However, she would only go to the hospital if it were in another state. She was paranoid and delusional. She appeared disheveled, there was inadequate food in the house, and the electric company was threatening to turn off her power for nonpayment of her bill. It took two days of attempts by the nurse to persuade Ms. R. to enter the hospital due to her physical and psychological condition. Mrs. R. was hospitalized, treated, and eventually returned home with continued follow-up at the community health center.

ADVOCACY

The rural elderly have been a forgotten segment of the population and need advocacy at the individual, community and national level.

Advocacy for the elderly has been enhanced by REOP in several ways. Individual advocacy is aimed at empowering clients in their use of the health or social care system, and to enhance patients' and families' self-reliance for self-care. At the community level, bringing the groups caring for the rural elderly together into a coalition has strengthened the power, visibility, and planning abilities of these organizations. Through work with various community groups and participation in public hearings on the health care needs of rural elderly, public attention has been focused on the plight of this population and the issues surrounding rural mental health delivery. Advocacy at the national level has included the preparation of briefing papers for congressional personnel, and presentations to national meetings and conferences. Advocacy also includes education. The clinical nurse specialists are involved in a number of community education efforts, including chairing the local health promotion coalition; providing articles for local newspapers; and presenting information on topics related to aging at local, state, and national forums.

Case Study–Ms. L.

Ms. L. is a 76-year old white widow who has a number of chronic health problems, including adult onset diabetes, atherosclerotic heart disease, congestive heart failure, congenital blindness of her right eye and cataracts. When first seen, Ms. L. was being followed by a local physician and a home health agency. She was having daily episodes consistent with hypoglycemia, which were often manifested by falling. The clinical nurse specialist was able to bring these problems to the attention of her health care providers, which led to hospitalization and readjustment of her hypoglycemic medication. Also through the advocacy of the nurse, Ms. L.'s cataracts were evaluated and removed. This surgery restored some of her vision and enabled her to enjoy activities which she thought were lost to her, such as reading and enjoying family photographs. Other advocacy efforts for Ms. L. have included working with the home health agency and social services agency to obtain a care aide, and with the area agency on aging to obtain home care equipment.

CONCLUSION

The rural elderly have been a neglected segment of the population. Their mental health care needs are great, but have been poorly met in the past. The program and methods described in this chapter represent an approach that has proven itself clinically successful in overcoming the multiple difficulties inherent in delivering care to the rural elderly with mental health problems. Although the program was designed to be appropriate for the rural southeast, its principles can be translated to other regions of the country, and can serve as a model to provide mental health care to this important segment of the "forgotten aged."

AUTHOR'S NOTE

This research was supported by grants from the W. K. Kellogg Foundation, the National Institutes of Health, the Pew Charitable Trusts, and the Division of Nursing of the U.S. Department of Health and Human Services. The opinions expressed in this chapter are those of the authors and do not necessarily reflect the views of the sponsors.

Address correspondence to: Diane G. Snustad, University of Virginia, Madison House, 170 Rugby Road, Charlottesville, VA 22903.

REFERENCES

Abraham, I. L., Buckwalter, K. C., Snustad, D. G., Smullen, D. E., Thompson-Heisterman, A. A., Neese, J. B., & Smith, M. (in press). Psychogeriatric outreach to rural families: The Iowa and Virginia models. *International Psychogeriatrics.*

Abraham, I. L. & Neese, J. B. (in press). Outreach to elderly and their families: Focus on the rural South. *Aging.*

Abraham, I. L., Neese, J. B., Buckwalter, K. C., Fox, J., Kane, C., & Turner, K. (under review). The mental health of minority and impoverished elderly in the rural South: Toward a research agenda.

Baker, F. M. (1988). Dementing illness and black Americans. In Jackson, J. S., *The black American elderly: Research on physical and psychosocial health* (pp. 215-236). New York: Springer.

Buckwalter, K. C., Abraham, I. L., Smith, M. A., & Smullen, D. E. (in press). Nursing outreach to mentally ill rural elderly. *Hospital and Community Psychiatry.*

Buckwalter, K. C., McLeran, H., Mitchell, S., & Andrews, P. H. (1988). Responding to mental health needs of the elderly in rural areas: A collaborative geriatric education center model. *Gerontology and Geriatrics Education*, 8(3/4), 69-80.

Buckwalter, K. C., Smith, M., Zevenbergen, P., Russell, D. (1991). Mental Health Services of the Rural Elderly Outreach Program. *The Gerontologist*, 31:3 (pp. 408-413).

Coward, R. T. & Lee, G. R. (1985). *The elderly in rural society: Every fourth elder*. New York: Springer Publishing Company.

Deprez, R. D., Pennell, B. E., & Libby, M. A. (1987). The substitutability of outpatient primary care in rural community health centers for inpatient hospital care. *Health Services Research*, 22, 207-233.

Fleming, A. A., Richardson, L. D., Santos, J. F., & West, P. R. (1988). Mental health services for elderly: Report on survey of community mental health centers. Vol. III. Washington, D.C.: Action Committee to Implement Mental Health Recommendations of the 1981 White House Conference on Aging.

George, L. K., Landerman, R., Blazer, D. G., & Anthony, J. C. (1991). Cognitive impairment. In L. N. Robins & D. A. Reiger, *Psychiatric disorders in America* (pp. 258-290). New York: Free Press.

Greene, V. L. (1984). Premature institutionalization among the rural elderly in Arizona. *Public Health Reports*, 99, 58-63.

Grusky, O. & Tierney, K. (1989). Evaluating the effectiveness of county wide mental health care systems. *Community Mental Health Journal*, 26, 3-20.

Harper, M. S. (1990). *Minority aging: Essential curriculum content for selected health and allied professionals*. Washington, D.C.: U.S. Government Printing Office.

Harper, M. S. & Alexander, C. D. (1990). Profile of the black elderly. In M.S. Harper (Ed.), *Minority aging: Essential curricula content for selected health and allied health professionals*. Washington, D.C.: U.S. Government Printing Office.

Human, J. & Wasem, C. (1991). Rural mental health in America. *American Psychologist*, 46, 240-243.

Jackson, J. S. (1988). *The black American elderly: Research on physical and psychosocial health*. New York: Springer.

Mandersheid, R. & Sonmenschein, M. A. (Eds.) (1990). *Mental health, United States 1990*. (DHHS Publication No. ADM 90-1708). Washington, D.C.: NIMH.

Neese, J. B., Abraham, I. L., Currie, L. J., Smullen, D., & Thompson-Heisterman, A. (1992). Rural elder program: Meeting health care needs. *Bridges*, 3(1), 2-3.

Palmore, E. (1983-84). Health care needs of the rural elderly. *International Journal of Aging and Human Development*, 18(1), 39-45.

President's Commission of Mental health (1978). Task Panel on Rural Mental Health (Vol. III, Appendix). Washington, D.C.: U.S. Government Printing Office.

Rosen, C. E., Coppage, S. J., Troglin, S. J., & Rosen, S. (1981). Cost effective mental health services for the rural elderly. In P. K. Kim & C. Wilson (Eds.),

Toward mental health of rural elderly. Washington, D.C.: University Press of America.

Scheidt, R. J. & Windely, P. G. (1982). Well-being profiles of small town elderly in differing rural contexts. *Community Mental Health Journal, 18,* 257-267.

Sommers, I. (1989). Geographic location and mental health services utilization among the chronically mentally ill. *Community Mental Health Journal, 25,* 132-144.

U. S. Congress, Office of Technology Assessment. (1990). *Health care in rural America.* (OTA-H-434). Washington, D.C.: U.S. Government Printing Office.

Wagenfeld, M. O. (1990). Mental health and rural America: A decade of review. *Journal of Rural Health, 6,* 507-522.

Waxman, H. M. (1986). Community mental health care for the elderly: A look at the obstacles. *Public Health Reports, 101,* 294-300.

Index

ABANDONMENT
  see loneliness
ACCESS
  see outreach
ACCULTURATION
  19
ADDICTION
  see alcohol
ADULT PROTECTIVE SERVICES
  42,
  see also outreach
AFFECTIVE DISORDER
  see depression,
    mania, Bradburn
AFRICAN-AMERICAN
  5-29,97,101,102,105,107
AGEISM
  66
AGGRESSION
  see anger
AGISM
  see ageism
AGITATION
  see anger
AIDS
  49
ALCOHOLISM
  50
ALZHEIMER'S DISEASE
  see dementia
ANGER
  63,68,73
ANIMALS
  see pets
ANOREXIA
  103,106
ANXIETY
  22,46,48,50,73,106
APPETITE
  see anorexia
ARTHRITIS
  106
ASSESSMENT of
  African Americans
    5-29
  dementia
    5-32,50,106
  depression
    11,15-29,65
  Hispanics
    15-29
  rural elders
    105-106

BDI
  17,26,27
BECK DEPRESSION INVENTORY
  17,26,27
BEREAVEMENT
  46,50,103,106
BIPOLAR DISORDER
  see mania
BLINDNESS
  see vision
BRADBURN AFFECT
  BALANCE SCALE 65
CANCER
  103,106
CARE DELIVERY
  see outreach
CAREGIVERS
  see family
CASE MANAGEMENT
  see outreach,
    psychotherapy
CASE STUDY dementia
  36-40
CASE STUDY depression
  99,101,105,106,107
CASE STUDY developmental
  disability 72-73,87-91
CASE STUDY rural elder
  99-108
CBS
  see dementia
CEREBRAL VASCULAR ACCIDENT
  101
CESD
  18,19,25,26,27
CHEMICAL DEPENDENCY
  see alcoholism
CHILDREN
  see family
CHRONIC BRAIN SYNDROME
  see dementia
CHURCH
  see religion
COGNITIVE IMPAIRMENT
  see dementia
COHABITATION
  see family
COHORT
  48,54
COMMUNITY, COMMUNITY ELDERS
  11,19,35,36-40
COMMUNITY SERVICES
  see outreach